Posture

How to Permanently Heal Your Posture Without Tons of Effort

(How Does Our Body Language Influence People Around Us)

Bret Sauter

Published By **Bella Frost**

Bret Sauter

Posture: How to Permanently Heal Your Posture Without Tons of Effort (How Does Our Body Language Influence People Around Us)

ISBN   978-1-998901-67-8

Legal & Disclaimer

The information contained in this book is not designed to replace or take the place of any form of medicine or professional medical advice. The information in this book has been provided for educational & entertainment purposes only.

The information contained in this book has been compiled from sources deemed reliable, and it is accurate to the best of the Author's knowledge; however, the Author cannot guarantee its accuracy and validity and cannot be held liable for any errors or omissions. Changes are periodically made to this book. You must consult your doctor or get professional medical advice before using any of the suggested remedies, techniques, or information in this book.

Table of Contents

Introduction 1

Chapter 1: Proven Techniques To Maintain Bone Strength 5

Chapter 2: The Ultimate Healing Yoga Poses 27

Chapter 3: Diagnostic Gymnastics (Checks) 44

Chapter 4: Balms That Provide Quick Relief 59

Chapter 5: How It Really Works Inside The Fight In Competition To Weight Issues... 68

Chapter 6: Yoga Tips For Beginners........ 80

Chapter 7: Bodyweight Exercises For The Chest/Back, Shoulders/Arms And Core!. 85

Chapter 8: The Psychology Of Change.... 93

Chapter 9: Standing Yoga Poses 106

Chapter 10: Strengthening Balance...... 119

Chapter 11: Breathing Tips When Running 124

Chapter 12: Postural Problems In The Child 141

Chapter 13: Borne Out Of Hinduism 157

Chapter 14: Beginning With Solving Your Posture 161

Chapter 15: Daily Habits Causing Bad Posture And How To Avoid Them 169

Chapter 16: Negative Effects Of Forward Head Posture 179

Conclusion 184

Introduction

This book consists of examined steps and strategies on a way to get started out with the workout of yoga and take benefit of the severa advantages it is able to provide. It competencies complete records on yoga and its severa blessings. Also blanketed on this book are practical suggestions on a way to get commenced with the exercising of yoga, some weight loss program tips similarly to three yoga etiquette to undergo in mind at the identical time as training yoga.

Yoga is described as an organized exercise of exercising, meditation, excessive pleasant questioning, healthy dietweight-reduction plan manage, relaxation and breath that's geared toward generating harmony inside the environment, thoughts and body. The practice of yoga entails low-effect physical actions, meditation, relaxation, respiratory techniques (known as pranayama) and poses (known as asanas). A lot of people are familiar with yoga positions regardless of the fact that most are not aware that the exercise of yoga consists of a lot more.

In the area of medicine, yoga techniques are being hired for the marketing of general health, in substance abuse treatment strategies as well as complementary treatment technique for ailments which incorporates HIV/AIDS, cancers, coronary heart issues, melancholy and anxiety troubles. The exercise of yoga is considered as a low-charge self-assist approach to commonplace nicely-being.

The word yoga is derived from the Sanskrit term "Yog", due to this union. Yoga is defined then as a union of the physical systems with the thoughts's popularity. In philosophy, yoga creates a union of energy (spirit or soul), thoughts and body to supply a nation of calmness or equanimity. Advancing greater, combining philosophy and generation, an person will revel in the union of internal electricity, thoughts, body and cosmic forces main to higher physical, intellectual fitness and in the long run self-recognition.

Some information of Yoga

The roots of yoga are rooted at a few stage inside the historical times in India. Yoga is a traditional device of highbrow and physical practices that originated in South Asia at a few degree in the Indus Valley civilization. The vital intention of yoga is to sell harmony within the mind, frame and the environment.

Yoga consists of a holistic device of social, mental, non secular and physical development. For over one thousand of years, the philosophies of yoga modified into exceeded on from the maintain close trainer to its university college students, it turned into round hundred BC while the very first written facts of the exercise of yoga first seemed in Yogasutra of Patanjali. The gadget of yoga includes the Asthangayoga or the eightfold route.

In Western nations, a number of yoga faculties are well-known and employs some or all of the limbs of Asthangayoga as described with the aid of Patanjali. Following are the 8 limbs:

1. Samadhi – final superior meditation techniques and psychic strategies achieved after the regular exercise for preferred attention

2. Dhyana – interest strategies for intellectual calmness and balance

three. Dhana – recognition techniques for intellectual calmness and stability

four. Pratihara – strategies for retaining apart the thoughts from the other senses to obtain intellectual calmness and balance

five. Pranayama – breathing strategies for highbrow and physical stability

6. Asaana – posture techniques for mental and physical stability that is what a whole lot of people understand as yoga.

7. Niyama – strategies for purifying and handling self

eight. Yama – pointers for effective and a achievement residing in community

Chapter 1: Proven Techniques To Maintain Bone Strength

When you keep robust bones even as you're despite the fact that greater youthful, your danger of getting bone-related headaches is decreased. As you age, you turn out to be more prone to fitness conditions like painful vertebral fractures on your spine. To help you decorate bone fitness, you could try the subsequent validated techniques:

• Get 5-10 minutes of solar publicity every day. Make it a addiction to spend some time out of doors to get your each day vitamins D.

• Consume cereal this is wealthy in diet D. Also, encompass fatty fish and eggs to your diet regime to enhance the quantity of food regimen D you get. Every day, you want at the least six hundred IU of this nutrition, or 800 IU for age 70 and beyond.

• Eat greater leafy greens, nuts, and beans. Pistachios, walnuts, and almonds are wealthy in calcium, which is good for the bones. For snacks, these nuts are exquisite options to get additional calcium. White beans and baked beans also are excellent property of calcium.

You can snack on them any time or add the nuts and beans on your desired soup. Leafy vegetables along aspect kale, bok Choy, and collard greens also contain calcium.

• Try a few canned salmon, shrimp, sardines, and unique seafood. These are packed with protein and calcium which might be important for bone health. If you want to get more omega-fatty acids, salmon is the notable deliver you may consider.

• Eat fortified oatmeal as a snack or for breakfast. Unsweetened on the spot oatmeal includes 100mg of calcium, this is type of 10% of the encouraged each day intake. Choose a emblem that gives greater vitamins without any introduced sugar. To improve calcium intake, you can consume your oatmeal with yogurt, almond milk, or entire milk.

• Stop smoking cigarettes. Bone loss is one of the crucial dangers of smoking. In addition, folks that smoke regularly have a horrible balance which makes them vulnerable to falling and getting a fractured bone.

• Go taking walks or walking each day. Although you may determine the frequency and pace of your jogs or walks, it's suitable to are looking for for recommendation out of your teacher or medical medical doctor about what's suitable. Generally, 20-half-hour in keeping with session and three-four times in keeping with week are distinctly recommended.

• Do jumping wearing activities, bench steps, or climb stairs. These bodily sports sports are specific alternatives to step up the intensity of your each day exercise from taking walks or taking walks. These exercises assist improve bones and achieve a more whole of lifestyles cardio exercising.

• Do power education. Pulling, pushing, and lifting weights 2-3 instances every week is an effective way to maintain bone strength and everyday fitness.

These strategies to hold healthful bones appear easy and smooth, but much less difficult said than executed. The primary secret's in your vicinity to comply with those recommendations and purpose them to part of your every day existence. Your manner of existence conduct extensively have an effect in your bone health as you age.

The properly facts is that there are natural strategies to ensure you're on the proper song to building healthy and sturdy bones. Check out the following smooth approaches to make each day an opportunity to decorate your bone power.

Eat More Veggies

This is a no-brainer, greens are accurate for the bones. They provide weight loss plan C that is vital in producing bone-forming cells within the course of the frame. According to analyze, the antioxidant homes of nutrients C help in defensive bones from mobile harm.

Moreover, vegetables furthermore assist in growing bone density to preserve it robust. Having low bone mineral density can result in brittle bones and coffee bone mass. These health situations placed you liable to getting bone illnesses which could negatively have an effect to your traditional properly-being.

For older women, ingesting veggies is more beneficial. A examine found that women age 50 and past who eat onions regularly are at 20%

lower chance of having brittle bones or osteoporosis, in assessment to girls who don't devour them. Another chance problem to endure in mind for older human beings is stepped forward bone turnover, a technique in which bones are broken right all of the way all the way down to shape a brand new bone.

Consuming extra than nine servings of parsley, cabbage, broccoli, and one-of-a-type veggies presents the body with bone-defensive antioxidants that lessen bone turnover. Therefore, it's vital to fill your plate with greens to construct healthy bone as you age.

Get Plenty of Vitamin K

Aside from food plan D, you furthermore may additionally additionally need to preserve up collectively along with your nutrients K each day intake. Vitamin K2, for instance, performs a important role in bone energy because it modifies osteocalcin to assist bone formation. This approach of trade allows osteocalcin to combine with minerals present within the bone to prevent calcium loss.

MK-four and MK-7 are not unusual varieties of nutrients K2. The former is observed in meat, eggs, and liver, even as the latter can be sourced from natto soybean merchandise, sauerkraut, cheese, and first rate fermented additives. According to 1 have a have a look at, taking MK-7 nutritional dietary supplements can help growth nutrients K2 blood levels better than MK-4.

However, taking any of the two varieties of weight-reduction plan K2 enables help osteocalcin change at the identical time as growing bone density in every located up-menopausal women and youngsters. Based on a observe, women many of the a long time of 50 to sixty five who take MK-4 dietary dietary supplements can hold bone density higher than those who gather a placebo.

Boost Zinc and Magnesium Intake

If you believe you studied calcium is the handiest mineral you must take to your bone health, then there a few thing you ought to recognize. Zinc and magnesium are also critical minerals to construct strong bones. Magnesium enables convert weight loss program D into an energetic shape in order that calcium is effortlessly absorbed through the body.

Most additives incorporate magnesium which makes supplementation a whole lot much less tough to manipulate. However, you may need to complement with magnesium carbonate, citrate, or glycinate to offer greater benefits in your bone health. Some super sources of magnesium embody pumpkin seeds, cashews, spinach, almonds, and peanuts.

Zinc is some different important hint mineral required to construct wholesome bones, however you only want a very small amount of this. It promotes bone-constructing mobile production while stopping too much breakdown of bones. According to studies, zinc supplements are effective in assisting a toddler's bone boom and keeping older an person's bone density.

Good hassle you could without problem encompass zinc in your each day diet regime through the usage of thinking about inclusive of spinach, pumpkin seeds, oysters, flax seeds, shrimp, and red meat for your food. You also can are looking for recommendation from your scientific medical doctor for the fantastic zinc nutritional supplements you may take if you're now not sure you're taking enough of this mineral out of your each day food regimen.

Simple Ways to Prevent Fractures

Have you ever been recognized with a fractured bone? A fracture or a damaged bone may be worrying and painful, specifically for children. Whether it's from a fall or an accident, it is able to recommend a few problems along with your bone's condition.

Luckily, there are smooth methods to avoid fractures. It all boils right right down to proper workout, weight loss plan, medicinal drugs, and assets to be had to you. Here are a few mind to prevent a damaged bone:

• Consult your fitness care company. In case you purchased into an twist of fate or a fall and broke a bone, it's essential to speak collectively along with your health care provider. They can help you decide the motives of the fracture, together with being related to osteoporosis.

Seeking expert recommendation is likewise useful in receiving the right clinical answer collectively with bone mineral density exam (DXA test). This is a technique to degree bone density in addition in your vulnerability to osteoporosis and other bone illnesses.

• Be extra careful. Preventing falls can be achieved with the useful resource of manner of without a doubt being careful at the same time as taking walks on slippery flooring or curbs. Always ensure to play it secure on the same time as you're outside. For instance, you may located on rubber footwear with suitable traction to keep away from falling which can result in a fracture. During lousy weather, older people can use a walker or cane in the event that they enjoy unstable.

When indoors, it's useful to preserve the floor muddle-free and use nightlights to make sure you don't experience whilst going to the toilet within the middle of the night. In addition, avoid walking round in floppy slippers or socks to prevent from slipping off. Place a rubber mat inside the tub or bathe ground to maintain yourself from falling at the same time as taking a shower.

Accidents can also additionally arise to human beings at any given time. However, being greater cautious can prevent from fractures and injuries. Make it a addiction to workout safety measures to maintain your bones in proper state of affairs.

Lifestyle Approaches for Better Bone Health

There are many things that human beings can do to promote bone health, from kids to antique age. Living a healthy way of life, as an instance, contributes an entire lot to an character's bone fitness, power, and normal fitness.

Since many minerals and vitamins are vital for your bone fitness, it's appropriate to eat a wholesome diet plan that includes components like cease result, greens, grains, beans, meat, calcium-rich ingredients, and espresso-fats dairy merchandise.

Most human beings in the United States don't take the encouraged degree of calcium in step with day, however ingesting the equal antique level is pretty viable. About three 8-ounce glasses of low-fat milk in keeping with day with a food plan containing calcium-rich meals are sufficient to get the encouraged level preferred thru the frame every day.

Elderly people don't get enough food regimen D from the sun. Therefore, it's crucial to take food plan D dietary supplements to enhance this vitamins degree for your frame together with a right weight loss plan. If you don't exit that hundreds to get some sun, taking dietary supplements is the super possibility for you.

Moreover, you need to exercising consultation or perform a few physical activities for as a minimum half-hour consistent with day to assemble and maintain bone mass as you age. For children, it's especially recommended to physical video games for at the least 60 mins in step with day to satisfy the same vintage guiding principle for physical sports.

People ought to are seeking out professional assist almost about having medical conditions related to bones and using drug treatments to address signs and symptoms. For girls, it's vital to are seeking for recommendation from their doctor if menstruation doesn't prevent for 3 months.

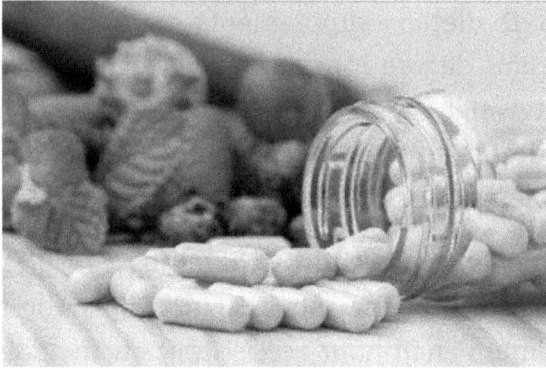

Bone-precise advice from the specialists can help you assemble a software program that works to your contemporary-day-day condition. You need to consist of the right physical sports activities sports further to nutrition so you can prevent numerous chronic illnesses inclusive of osteoporosis.

If you are lactose intolerant, there are a few tips to help you get enough calcium however your situation. You can pick dairy merchandise and calcium-rich additives that contain less lactose. For example, you can consume yogurt with stay bacteria that assist digest the lactose more effects.

Parmesan, Swiss, Colby, cheddar, and special difficult cheeses help in breaking down the lactose. In addition, lactose-reduced and lactose-free products which embody milk without lactose also are quality options. Then you can slowly increase the components you consume that encompass lactose.

Nutrients that you obtain from herbal materials are an entire lot better than dietary dietary supplements as they offer all of the essential minerals had to shield bone tissues. On the alternative hand, food dietary supplements also are amazing for people who can't devour sufficient calcium-rich components to satisfy the endorsed diploma consistent with day.

When it entails physical sports activities, the subsequent are some guidelines regarding the kind, period, intensity, and frequency of workout you want to sell bone electricity:

• It's important to make a lifelong determination to doing workout and physical hobby to virtually stimulate bones, muscle tissues, and splendid characteristics of health.

• Creativity and variety are important to keep doing physical sports sports in the long run.

• Exercises and different bodily sports tremendously have an effect on the skeletal bones which can be loaded or compelled by way of the sports. Meaning, wearing occasions don't advantage your whole skeleton, however they may provide a few blessings to bone health in location of doing not whatever in any respect.

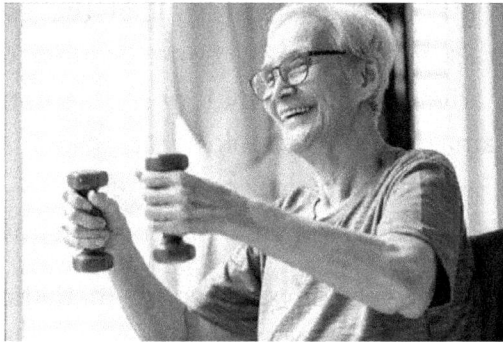

• Bone benefit can display up at the same time as the stimulus is greater than the conditions your bones commonly enjoy. However, applying static masses constantly like fame doesn't assist growth bone mass.

• A extended period of immobility and shortage of physical activities can motive bone loss. If you may't keep away from being immobile which encompass even as you're unwell and want to relaxation, you can perform a short weight-bearing exercise to reduce bone loss.

• Daily physical activity which includes stability-improving, strength-building, and weight-bearing bodily video games instances or more instances everyday with week considerably growth bone strength.

• Any sports that encompass impact which encompass skipping and jumping can assist growth bone density in desire to low- to mild-depth sports like brisk on foot. Endurance sports activities additionally help boom muscle groups, coordination, and balance on the equal time as preventing falls in older humans.

• Jumping and other load-bearing physical games don't need to take longer to get the advantages to bone power. You can perform at least 5-10 mins of lengthy-bearing physical activities each day. Ideally, you may begin with weight-bearing physical sports and slowly add jumping and skipping bodily video games in your regular.

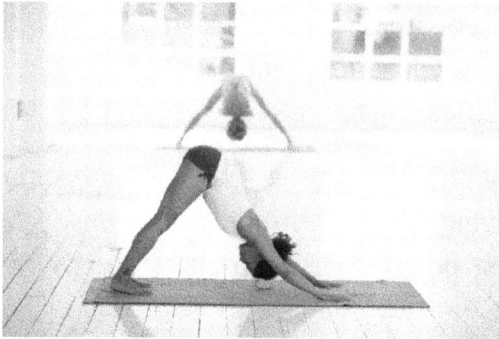

On the opportunity hand, weight training, further to taking walks and on foot, may additionally want longer durations along with 30-forty five mins to get effects. If you've been inactive for a while, it's essential to observe this encouraged time and frequently use a modern-day-day plan.

For example, start with clean bodily video video games with short times like on foot or mild weights. Every week, boom the depth or time via 10% to keep away from fractures or accidents.

• Physical sports activities like aerobic training and strength education can help bone mass higher than doing carrying sports that contain normal or everyday loading styles like walking.

As you age, it's turning into even extra difficult to preserve up with bone fitness. When you're

60 years antique and beyond, fall prevention moreover turns into important to avoid intense bone accidents which might be typically difficult to restore in the course of vintage age.

How to Prevent Falls

More frequently than no longer, falls are the cause of fractures in particular in people with lower bone mineral density. Preventing falls is a notable manner to lessen your risk of bone harm. Falls commonly motive fractures inside the hip, pinnacle arm, pelvis, wrist, and spine.

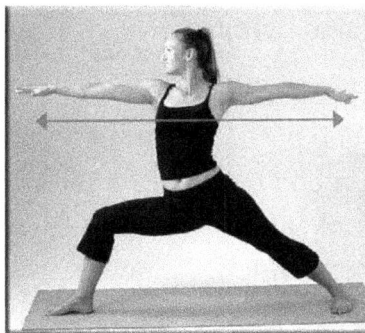

Various factors cause falls, consequently prevention strategies ought to be superior based totally on the ones more than one components. Aside from doing bodily sports sports, there are one of a type techniques to reduce your chances of falling or lower effect in case it happens to you. Check out the subsequent:

• Whether it's extreme or not, it's vital to allow your healthcare issuer recognize about the fall you've had. Usually, businesses test up on their patients as quickly as a year to look if there are problems due to falls or accidents.

• Get your healthcare issuer to have a examine you for balance or your functionality to walk if you've fallen once or numerous instances. This is crucial to keep away from a extra intense scientific hassle that may be as a result of a neglected minor damage.

• Fall evaluation is needed for those who skilled falls within the past 12 months. The assessment includes how and even as the fall occurred and a take a look at of stability, coronary heart characteristic, vision, blood strain, muscle energy, and walking. A geriatrician or related professional will conduct this evaluation.

• Healthcare groups ought to be able to prescribe a application that includes stability education and physical sports activities to their sufferers. Physical sports activities ought to attention on decreasing the risk of falling.

• Patients must have their medicinal drugs reviewed via their healthcare corporations earlier than taking them in conjunction with OTC medicines as soon as a 365 days. This allows save you treatment problems that might result in falls which consist of better doses of medicine and drug-to-drug interactions.

• Vision test-americashould be finished as quickly as a 365 days.

• Home evaluation should be finished for capacity dangers that can purpose falls consisting of electrical cords, awful lighting fixtures, unfastened rugs, and shortage of handrail inside the bathe or bathtub.

• Be greater cautious even as the usage of ladders, ensure they're robust in advance than stepping on them. Step ladders with handrails also are better to apply than the ones without manual.

Other techniques to prevent falls are to position on hip pads or hip protectors to lessen your chance of fracture, particularly in case you're residing in an institutionalized care setting. Falls don't frequently mean you're aging, they may be normally due to each day physical sports activities sports and distinctive factors that placed you susceptible to falling.

To help you manage an twist of future-free environment, a few vital matters must be taken into consideration. For example, decluttering your home is the quality way to keep away from tripping over on footwear, garments, books, papers, and one of a kind unorganized subjects. Instead of using throw rugs, you could use rubber mats or use double-sided tape to hold your rugs from transferring or slipping.

Keep your gadgets in an smooth-to-access cupboard, so there's no want to use a step stool to get some thing. Put handrails or snatch bars for your bathe or bathtub to keep away from falling from the slippery ground. As you age, it's vital to improve your property lighting fixtures. Brighter lights can help avoid slip-offs at the same time as frosted bulbs and lampshades help lessen glare.

Aside from having your medicinal capsules reviewed through way of way of your healthcare issuer, it's moreover a need to to go through a vision test. An eye professional must take a look at your eyes as carrying beside the point glasses can smash your imaginative and prescient. In addition, having cataracts, glaucoma, and unique conditions can restrict your imaginative and prescient. Falls are the result of having bad vision.

Cases of falling usually boom sooner or later of much less warm months because of shorter days, snow, and ice. And the most debilitating falls frequently appear at domestic at some level inside the night time as human beings upward push up to answer the smartphone or visit the rest room. Therefore, watch out for cellar stairs with out handrails, shoes, or slippers that don't have rubberized pads or soles, sick-placed quantities of furniture, and slim passages with contortions or twists.

Following the ones pointers on bodily sports activities, way of life behaviors, and food regimen permit you to obtain proper bone fitness. After all, the goal is to reap senior age with strong and healthy bones as it's a extremely good element on your freedom to transport while you switch out to be vintage. So, what do you receive as real with you studied is the final change which you need to do for your manner of life to hold bone strength?

Chapter 2: The Ultimate Healing Yoga Poses

With the passing days, more and more studies is demonstrating that Yoga and meditation offer big benefits to folks who revel in the unwell outcomes of persistent illnesses. This is not to indicate that Yoga will treatment a long haul or persistent ailment, however if it's far observed as a dependable recurring, Yoga can manipulate some of illnesses through reducing anxiety, decreasing manifestations of the diseases, and facet effects of prescription, boosting the immune framework, and helping in wellknown fitness and modern solace. Here is a listing of effective Yoga asanas to remedy you from persistent ache:

Mountain pose (Tadasana):

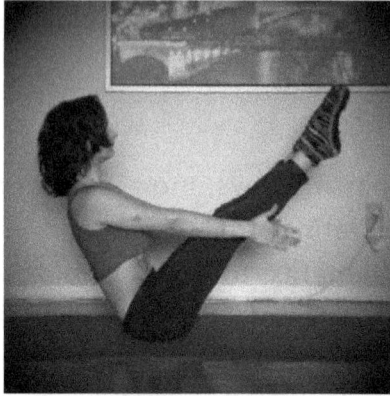

This asana is quite smooth to take a look at up and is protected inside the easy asanas of Yoga. In a standing feature, keep your ft apart and raise your toes. Then pull your knee caps as a good deal as thighs. Inhale and look up at the same time as doing so. While exhaling drop the shoulders and returned and gently press your top frame to the wall. Align yourself into an "H" position, breathing at maximum 8 times after which launch.

Benefits

• Reduces decrease once more pain

• Strengthens muscle corporations of thighs, stomach, and buttocks

• Improves hobby

• Relieves strain and sciatica

Tree pose (Vriksasana):

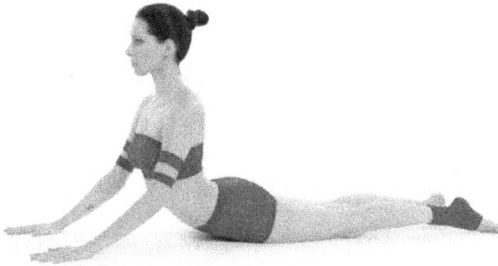

This asana begins with bending your right foot and placing it on your left thigh. Keeping your left leg regular, fold your hands above your head and examine item, then preserve a steady gaze. Breathe slowly and hold the posture for short time. Then repeat with the opportunity leg.

Benefits

• Rejuvenates the entire body

• Stretches arms, legs and lower lower back

• Improves attention

Straight ahead bend (hastapadasana):

Balancing your complete frame weight on every your feet, expand your palms overhead while breathing in. Slowly exhale and whilst exhaling bend beforehand down inside the path of your feet. Remain within the posture for approximately 30 seconds and maintain taking deep breathes. With regaining your posture, breathe in and stretch your fingers upwards and are to be had again to the recognition posture.

Benefits

• Increases bloody deliver eventually of the frame

• Spine receives supple

• Stretches and strengthens all the muscle groups in the decrease again

Warrior Pose (Veerbhadrasana):

This warrior pose starts offevolved with tadasana. Keep your leg as a minimum four ft aside. Turning your left toes with the beneficial useful resource of about 15 stages and proper foot by using using 90, stretch your palms massive. Lift your hands on your shoulder pinnacle. With palm coping with upwards, breathe out and bend your right knee. Turning your head, keep a regular gaze closer to your proper. Gently push your pelvis down and function smile of a warrior. Exhaling, stand up. Repeat the identical positions with the opposite element as nicely.

Benefits

• Highly useful for frozen shoulders

• Increases stamina and equilibrium of the body

• An powerful pressure removal Yoga asana

• Useful for people with desk jobs

Bridge pose (Setubandhasana)

Unlike one-of-a-kind positions, this one starts offevolved offevolved offevolved with mendacity flat in your decrease again. Fold your knees and maintain your ft apart like 12 inches far from your pelvis. Your knees and ankles need to be in a immediately line. Place your fingers beside your body, arms touching the floor. Inhaling gently, increase your decrease once more, then center and then higher returned rolling inside the shoulders. Slowly contact the chest to your chin with out shifting your chin. Keep your thighs parallel to the floor and experience your bottom agency up because of the pose. With smooth breathes, preserve the posture for about a minute and release lightly. You can also use your palms to assist your decrease lower back.

Benefits

• Relaxes a worn-out yet again

• Reduces tension and strain

• Increases decrease lower back muscle strength

• Opens up air passages and allows with thyroid issues.

• Also allows with digestion.

Butterfly pose (bandhakonasana)

Sit on a mat, unfold your legs out and all over again directly. Bending your knees, convey your ft to your pelvis as near as viable. Also your soles of the feet ought to be touching each one-of-a-kind. You can location your palms under your feet for manual after which clutch your toes tightly. Inhale deeply; begin flapping your legs like wings. Make fine to start with your begin gradual then growth your velocity. Try flying better and maintain your inhaling check. As you flap, your muscle tissues will will be inclined to loosen up. Taking a deep breath will supply your torso up. Exhale and unfold your legs to relax.

Benefits

• Helps bowel and intestine actions

• Improves flexibility of the hip, legs, and groin place

• Removes fatigue

• Helps with menstrual pain and menopause

• Smoothens transport if finished often

Thunderbolt pose (Vajrasana)

Another incredible simple asana however enormously beneficial is vajrasan. First of all fold your legs, placing your hips on the heels, sit down down on the little pit-type formation regular with the aid of your toes. Keeping your posture erect and head right now, vicinity your hands in your thighs and hold the posture and breathe deeply. Slowly lighten up and then straighten out your legs.

Benefits

• Food gets digested well in case you take a seat on vajrasan after having your meals.

• Blood circulate is stepped forward inside the decrease abdomen place

• Helps with diabetes, gastric and some specific belly associated pains

• Helps in stopping nice rheumatic ailments.

• Helps in meditation and keeps spine erect and the posture up right.

• Relaxes legs and decrease again muscle businesses

Sitting half of spinal twist (Ardha matsyendrasana)

Sit up with the legs prolonged right away in advance than you, keeping the toes collectively and the spine erect. Bend the left leg and positioned the heel of the left foot along the right hip (as an alternative, you can maintain the left leg right away). Take the right leg over the left knee. Then area your left hand on the proper knee and the right hand at the back of you. Twist the middle, shoulders and neck on this way to one side and appearance over the proper shoulder. Keep the spine erect. Hold and continue with easy prolonged breaths outside and inside. Breathing out, discharge the proper hand first (the hand within the back of you), discharge the stomach, then chest, in the end the neck and sit up straight free however immediately. Repeat to the subsequent issue. Breathing out, cross back to the front and unwind.

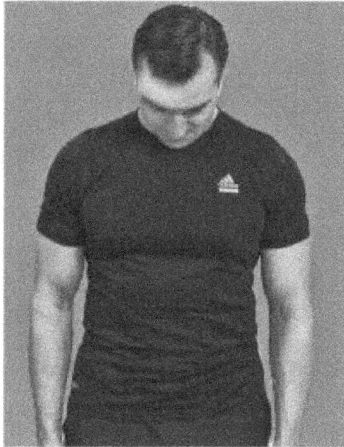

Benefits

• Spines stays supple

• Spinal elasticity is progressed

- Air passage to the lungs is opened and will growth air inlet to the lungs.

The boat pose (Naukasana)

Lie in your again collectively collectively together with your feet collectively and palms adjacent in your frame. Take a entire breath in and as you breathe out, deliver your mid-phase and ft off the floor, extending your arms in the direction of your ft. Your eyes, hands and toes ought to be in a line. Feel the anxiety on your navel area as the stomach muscle corporations settlement. Keep respiration profoundly and outcomes at the same time as maintaining up the stance. As you breathe out, go back to the ground step by step and unwind.

Benefits

- Helps toning up arm and leg muscle companies

- Back and stomach muscle businesses are strengthened

- Quite beneficial for hernia humans

Cobra pose (Bhujang asana)

Lying down on your stomach, maintain your feet leveled with the ground and temple touching the ground. Join the legs near every distinctive; lightly permit your heel and ft touching each one in all a type. Rest your palms beneath your shoulders, your elbows resting parallel and close to your higher frame. Taking an entire breath in, grade by grade increase your head, mid-section and stomach location on the identical time as maintaining your navel on the floor. Pulling your middle again up and then lifting it off the ground with the aid out of your arms. Keep your respiration technique with mindfulness, as you bend your backbone vertebra with the useful aid of vertebra. In the occasion that manageable, straighten your fingers with the aid of the usage of curving your decrease decrease lower back but loads as have to fairly be anticipated; tilt your head lower lower back and gaze upward. Relaxing your shoulders casually, if desired you could barely bend your elbows. With not unusual exercise, you could have the ability to increase the stretch through straightening the elbows. Make positive that your feet are near to three distinctive. Don't overcompensate the stretch or turn out to be overstraining yourself.

Exhaling slowly, delicately take your guts, mid-section and lie at the floor.

Benefits

• Eases up frozen shoulders and neck

• Strengthens the once more muscle corporations and shoulders

• Increases elasticity of the returned.

• Widens up the chest

• Increases blood skip

• Helps human beings dwelling with respiratory or lung related ailments.

Bee breath (Bhramari pranayama)

To carry out this pranayama, one ought to sit down immediately in a snug characteristic with eyes shut. Ensure the location you chose to perform the asana is properly-ventilated. Once you agree down within the function, area the tips on the ears and forefingers on the ligament that is placed some of the ears and cheeks. Take deep breathe in and on the equal time as you exhale, press the ligament. While you lightly press this ligament, make a murmuring sound like a bee – a low pitch sound.

Benefits

• Instantaneous stress, anger and tension reliever.

• Follows up a very effective respiratory approach and calms humans with excessive blood pressure.

• Spares you from an unpleasant headache

• Improves reminiscence and awareness

• Helps with migraines

• Helps with blood stress and controls it.

Sun salutation (Surya namaskar)

To do the proper Surya namaskar, those are the steps you want to comply with:

#1 Pranamasana (Prayer posture)

Join your toes together thru status toward the stop of your mat. Then balance your weight on each of your toes equally. Expand your chest and ease up your shoulders. As you inhale, enhance your fingers in your thing. While exhaling, be a part of your palms, as even though saluting, in the the front of your chest.

#2: Hastauttanasana (Raised arms pose)

While inhaling deep, increase your hands above your head excessive and hold your hands near the ears. Maintaining this posture, the exertion is to boom the complete body up from the fingertip to ft. You also can push the pelvis and lean in advance a tiny bit. Guarantee you are coming to up with the fingertips in place of attempting to bend in reverse.

#three: Hasta Padasana (Hand to foot pose)

Exhaling, bend down from your waist, your spine need to be erect. As you breathe out absolutely, convey your palms right all the way down to the ground, next to the feet. Bending your knees is non-compulsory, fundamental if you want it, to touch the ground at the side of your hands. Presently venture to preserve your knees erect. It's a clever concept to recuperation your palms settled within the palm- touching- floor function and maintain it till you complete the succession.

#four: Ashwa Sanchalanasana (Equestrian pose)

For this asana, you want to push your right leg as another time as possible. Then contact your proper knee to the ground and gaze upward.

Please take a look at that your left foot is exactly inside the center of the hands.

#5:Danda asana (Stick pose)

Breathing in, stretch your left leg back and preserve it beside your proper leg and preserve your posture without delay. For help you may region your palm on the ground.

#6:Ashtanga Namaskara (Salute with 8 sections)

Tenderly touch the floor alongside side your knees and breathe out. Pushing your hips decrease lower back specifically lay in advance, relaxation your chin and torso at the ground. Lift your lower returned a tad bit and the 2 ft, arms, knees, mid-phase and jaw (eight sections of the frame touch the floor).

#7: Bhujangasana (Cobra pose)

Move ahead and lift your torso up into main into the Cobra pose. If desired, you may maintain your elbows bowed in this represent, the shoulders an extended way out of your ears. Turn upward as you breathe in, try and push the mid-phase in advance; as you breathe out, pushing your navel down. Guarantee you are extending the identical quantity of strain as a whole lot as you can; do not stress your frame.

#eight: Parvat asana (Mountain pose)

Exhaling deeply, decorate your hips and tail bone immoderate, mid-phase driven down in an 'altered V' (/) stance. In the event this is feasible, try and attempt touching the floor at the side of your heels and try to your tailbone immoderate, going further into the posture of inverted V.

#nine: Ashwa Sanchalanasana (Equestrian pose)

Inhaling, convey your proper foot in amongst your fingers resting on the ground, left knee touching the floor, pushing your hips down and turn upward.

#10: Hasta Padasana (Hand to foot pose)

Exhaling, boom your foot, the left one. Let your palms be regular to the floor. If crucial, bend your knees. Tenderly straighten the knees and on the off hazard that you could, strive and strive touching your nose to the knees. Continue breathing.

#eleven: Hasta uttanasana (Raised palms pose)

Inhaling, beautify your torso up, enhance your hands and allow them to bend backwards, pushing the hips marginally outward.

#12: Tada asana (standing right away pose)

While breathing out, hold your posture uptight after which slide your arms to your aspect. Unwind in this role; experience and pay interest the slight feelings at some point of your frame.

It's trusted that large portions of those advantages are an instantaneous after impact of Yoga's accentuation on respiratory and centering the psyche, which moreover diminishes a part of the intellectual hassle that goes with lengthy haul contamination.

Chapter 3: Diagnostic Gymnastics (Checks)

I endorse you, before the begin of training with isometric gymnastics, to undergo the unique checking out in the form of easy physical games. This gymnastics will assist to attract your interest to the presence of wonderful troubles in wonderful elements of the spine and joints, if you have any.

Test of mobility in the cervical (neck) spine

Standing in front of the mirror, check the quantity and freedom of motion in the cervical backbone with the useful resource of bending your head earlier so, that your chin reaches on your chest. If that is tough, then there is a restrict of flexion of the cervical backbone.

Turn your head first to at least one and then to the opposite issue in order that the nose is flush with the shoulder. The problem of this movement well-knownshows a limit of rotation within the cervical backbone.

After that, tilt your head decrease again, directing your gaze upwards. If your chin rises to the quantity of your finger and better than it

- with the extension of the cervical spine you are all proper.

Restrictions in flexion, extension or rotation inside the cervical backbone can be associated with osteochondrosis of the backbone, the advent of a herniated disc, arthrosis of the spinal joints or rheumatic inflammatory technique within the backbone. In each of those instances, expert advice is wanted.

Mobility test in the thoracic (higher back) spine

Starting role: reputation with ft shoulder-width aside. You need an assistant to perform this take a look at. In the center of the thoracic backbone, your assistant have to feel the bone protrusion of one spinous technique with a finger and mark it on the pores and pores and skin with a marker.

Next, he should retreat down three spinous strategies and moreover mark them. Then you slowly lean earlier and down. If at some point of a dishonest your assistant sees how the spinous techniques skip apart and the gap among the marks will growth, the mobility of the vertebrae is ordinary.

If at some stage in numerous tries the distance among the marks does not alternate, there may be a limit of mobility in the thoracic backbone.

Mobility take a look at in the lumbar (lower again) backbone

Starting feature: repute with ft shoulder-width apart.

Feel the bony protrusions of the spine within the midline of the loin collectively together with your arms - those are spinous approaches of the vertebrae.

Place the second and third palms of 1 hand at the adjoining spinous techniques.

Holding your fingers on the spine, you ought to slowly lean in advance and down. If throughout the inclination you experience how the spinous strategies float aside and the distance among the arms will growth, the mobility of the vertebrae is regular. If for the duration of numerous attempts the distance does not change and also you do now not experience discrepancies within the vertebrae - feasible, there is a limit of mobility inside the lumbar spine.

Limiting the mobility of the lumbar vertebrae may be a final results of inflammatory lesions of the backbone and require treatment from a rheumatologist.

Hypermobility syndrome (prolonged flexibility) diagnosis check of joints

Try without try to pass the proposed test. If you score 6 and more elements, you can have an progressed mobility (hypermobility) of the joints. In this case, the traditional gymnastics, stressing the joints, you want to do with warning and handiest after consulting a medical doctor. The most quantity of things is nine.

Attention! A wholesome man or woman with normal mobility within the joints will now not be capable of skip this take a look at.

• Extend the little finger via way of 90 ° (1 thing for each hand, Fig. A).

• Bring your thumb sooner or later of the component and decrease again till it touches the forearm (1 aspect for every hand Fig. B).

• Bend the elbow joint via 10 ° (1 factor for every arm, Fig. C).

• Bend your knee by manner of 10 ° (1 problem for each leg, Fig. D).

• Touch your palms to the ground with out bending your knees (1 component, Fig. E).

Hypermobility (multiplied mobility) of the joints may be accompanied with the resource of the use of an improved threat of subluxation and different joint accidents, osteoarthritis and musculoskeletal ache with the formation of painful factors and nodes in the place of the bone protrusions. This circumstance is taken into consideration even as diagnosing and prescribing treatment, together with physiotherapy sports.

Isometric gymnastics appears to be existence-saving for the patient with hypermobility of the joints and it's far tremendously useful as it avoids injuries to the joints, which may be a susceptible issue from delivery in such sufferers and on the same time strengthens the muscle organizations and concurrently the ligaments.

Fibromyalgia (muscle pain) self-evaluation take a look at

Fibromyalgia syndrome may be a purpose of not unusual generalized ache - "it hurts everywhere". Often it is combined with low mood and fatigue and calls for a very precise approach within the training of a treatment software.

• Moderately squeeze the muscle roller of the trapezius muscle with 1 and a pair of fingers (see on Fig.). You ought to do it on every sides: left and proper.

Press on stage of second rib on every factor of the sternum like on photo.

Push down the fats pad at the inner of every knee like on picture.

The presence of excessive ache in all of these factors may additionally moreover indicate a likely presence of fibromyalgia.

You can independently suspect fibromyalgia in your self, however simplest a scientific medical health practitioner, typically a rheumatologist, can installation this analysis. Fortunately, no matter the as an alternative painful manifestations of this situation, the affected person does not find out any signs and symptoms of excessive inflammatory or degenerative harm to the joints or muscle groups. And given that muscular tissues are the number one intention for this sickness, they need to be treated.

Do not expect that banal physical training, walking or health can assist solve this kind of problem to all sufferers. These people be via using actual ache and cannot tolerate heavy bodily exertion. Therefore, you ought to load the muscle organizations and joints metered. Choose from an isometric gymnastics complicated the ones sports activities that have an impact in your most painful muscle businesses. Let them turn out to be a part of your normal training, every for the reason of remedy and for the prevention of exacerbation of the illness.

Test that the length of your legs is equal

Lie on a flat ground, bend the knee joints as a lot as 90 °, and be a part of the toes collectively. It is important to precisely align the heels and thumbs (for accuracy, you could use your thumbs to rest towards a wall or vertical floor popularity next to it). Look on the pleasant factor of the contour of the knee - if the point of 1 knee is decrease, it's far possible that this leg is shortened.

The shortening of the leg may be absolute, even as the bones of 1 leg are absolutely shorter than the opportunity, or relative, at the same time as the period of the bones is identical, but due to the pelvic misalignment, one leg is better and is functionally longer. In the case of a massive shortening, it could be important to in particular accurate the insole or shoes.

Test the arch of the foot - do you have have been given flat toes?

Wet foot print check:

On a easy, dry and preferably dark floor, leave a print with a wet foot. Evaluate your mark and determine how cited is the arch of the foot.

a) the arch of the foot is mild, you've got had been given flat feet;

b) the arch of the foot is normal;

c) the arch of the foot is just too said.

Too susceptible arch (flat-footedness) or excessively advised arch of the foot motives ache inside the foot and adjacent joints (together with the knee). This regularly shows concomitant systemic sicknesses and may require using orthopedic insoles or footwear.

Determine the power of your feet

Try to walk on feet after which on heels. If you have had been given enough power to carry out severa steps in the ones positions, the muscle agencies and nerves that control the feet feature normally. If one foot falls within the back of and is in reality weaker in any role, then it's far very possibly that there may be muscle prone issue, that is, partial paralysis.

Difficulties in strolling on toes or heels can be associated with muscle weak point (paresis or partial paralysis). The maximum common reason of such weak point is a hernia of the lumbar intervertebral disc, which squeezed the nerve root. Less usually, this is because of harm to the peripheral nerve. Paresis or paralysis of the foot calls for session with a neurologist or a neurosurgeon.

Test the knee joint - what sound do you listen?

Starting function: reputation with ft shoulder-width apart. Slowly squat, bending the legs at the knee joints in half of, repeat the squat severa times. If this movement is achieved with out trouble and your knee joints make no sounds, you're in ideal order. If during a squat you pay hobby a creak or superb sounds - problems are just throughout the corner. If the squeak is observed through ache - the problem is apparent.

The cartilaginous surfaces of the knee joints are below exceptional stress; consequently, they're the primary to respond with sound at some point of degenerative lesions due to arthrosis. Painful squeaks in the knee joints reflect the growing older of cartilage, which requires observation and treatment.

Test how loads fluid inside the knee joint

Sit on a chair, straighten your knee simply. Feel for the kneecap. Grip the knee together with your proper hand simply so the thumb pushes the joint tissue on one facet and the possibility 4 fingers on the alternative; patella can be amongst them. Press lightly together together with your palms on the joint tissue. With the thumb of your left hand, press down on the middle of the kneecap. If there can be an excess amount of fluid in the joint, the kneecap will go together with the waft in it and knock elastically at the bones to be underneath it. If the quantity of fluid is everyday, then the kneecap will stay tightly pressed towards the bones and you'll not pay attention a knock.

Excess fluid inside the knee joint can also advise inflammation or trauma. This condition always calls for professional advice.

Test the us of a of your hip joints

In the supine function, bend the test leg at the knee joint and area the heel on the alternative knee joint. Now slowly lower the knee joint to the side. At this 2nd there can be a rotation within the hip joint. Normally, you may be capable of decrease the knee nearly to the horizontal degree without large problem. The limit of this movement shows a likely pathology of the hip joint.

Rotation within the hip joint is impaired widely speakme due to arthrosis. The appearance of a restriction of rotation inside the hip joint most often speaks of the onset of the illness and requires orthopedic consultation.

Test the circumstance of the shoulder joints

First area each hands at the decrease lower back of the pinnacle, and then vicinity the arms within the decrease back of your returned, setting them at the lower once more. If there aren't any issues inside the shoulder joints, then the ones actions are completed results and in entire. The restriction of those moves shows a possible lesion of the shoulder joints.

Bend the arm beneath check on the elbow to a proper attitude and squeeze the brush into a fist. Press your elbow to your frame. Holding the elbow on the body, push the fist out. At this second there may be a rotation of the humerus inside the shoulder joint. Normally, you may pull the fist to forty five°. If the quantity of motion is hundreds much less - there can be pathology of the shoulder joint.

Limiting the rotation of the shoulder also can recommend pathology of the shoulder joint, most customarily because of infection, rupture or scarring of the joint tablet or the tendons of the rotator cuff. This scenario requires session with an orthopedist. As a rule, this kind of affected individual infrequently places his fingers in the back of his another time or at the back of his head. This reasons big issues in ordinary life and self-care, as it turns into difficult to get dressed, wash, brush hair.

Check the elbow joints

Hold any object firmly in the brush. If pains inside the elbow joints seem, there can be infection in this location.

Bend the tested arm inside the elbow joint to a right attitude and turn the brush with the back component up. Exercise stress behind the hand at the opportunity arm, which prevents extension of the wrist. In case of infection in the external epicondyle of the elbow joint, you will revel in pain there.

Now turn the hand beneath check with the palm up. Similarly, observe strain with the palm of your hand on the other arm, which prevents flexion in the wrist joint. In case of inflammation in the inner epicondyle of the elbow joint, you'll enjoy pain there.

Inflammation of the outside epicondyle (outdoor epicondylitis, or "tennis player's elbow") or internal epicondyle (internal epicondylitis, or "swimmer's elbow") is manifested usually while walking with a broom or at some point of direct strain on those regions. Treatment of this situation takes numerous months and requires the intervention of a consultant.

Test carpal tunnel syndrome

Align the rear of each fingers and area them in the the front of the chest, with the hands pointing down, and every forearm and hand shape a proper mind-set. Press the brushes lightly in opposition to every one-of-a-kind and keep this role for 1 minute. If you have had been given carpal tunnel syndrome, you can enjoy pain, numbness or tingling on your palms and hands within the path of this time.

The narrowing of the canal inside the wrist vicinity, wherein the median nerve passes, motives pain, numbness and painful goosebumps in the arms and forearms, disrupting each ordinary performance and night rest. This scenario is handled by the usage of both conservative and surgical strategies.

Check the temporomandibular (jaw) joint

Open your mouth substantial. Normally, you could freely positioned 3 of your hands, mendacity on pinnacle of every distinctive, into the mouth. Move your chin backward and forward.

Limiting the outlet of the mouth within the sort of position or lateral actions of the jaw, the advent of ache or unsightly clicks sooner or later of those moves might also suggest pathology of the temporomandibular (jaw) joint.

Overall posture evaluation

Evaluate your posture in a tall replicate, looking at your self straight away and to the thing. Pay hobby to the height and symmetry of the shoulders, the symmetry of the determine as a whole, the splendor and smoothness of the curves of the backbone. Explicit defects of posture will right now attraction to your interest. Consult in this example at the clinical medical doctor.

Chapter 4: Balms That Provide Quick Relief

When flare-u.S.In your decrease again arise, speedy consolation can by no means be close to sufficient. Here are a few natural home-made balm remedies that you can create and rub proper in to the ones hassle spots. Often someone can't wait to put together a tea to drink and as an alternative goals a quicker solution. Sometimes pills and extraordinary treatment may additionally take too lengthy to begin taking walks too. This is one of the many advantages of the use of balms due to the fact you could create them earlier of time, they're portable, and you could maintain them for pretty some time for long-term utilization.

#1 Balm - Cayenne Warming Balm

When searching out the elements to create an effective balm for back pain, we have decided that cayenne virtually works well. This pepper is identified as a remarkable healer whether or not or no longer or now not you use it within the body or on the out of doors. For this motive, you could use it inner a balm similarly to a tea, but you'll discover that once finished immediately for your lower once more, it will artwork faster and plenty greater efficaciously. The warm temperature will will let you loosen up factors of your muscle mass hastily, that could offer a short method to the ache in your once more. Keep in mind that this balm won't be for absolutely everyone, so make certain to check it in a small location in advance than rubbing it all through. Make high excellent to clean each arms after the use of and make sure not to get it for your face as it could motive a burning sensation for your eyes or nose.

Ingredients:

1. ½ cup of more virgin olive oil

2. ½ ounce of grated beeswax

three. 2 teaspoons of cayenne powder

Directions:

1. Using a double boiler, combo together the olive oil and beeswax. Stir it collectively over a low hearth sincerely so it mixes collectively. Make fantastic to maintain stirring so it does now not start to burn.

2. Sprinkle on your cayenne powder similarly all through the beeswax/olive oil aggregate and stir.

three. Remove from the hearth and pour into your desired packing containers to allow cool. A tin can or glass jar that you could seal tightly is good. Rub into sore areas to your lower lower back.

#2 Balm – Cooling Balm

As an possibility to the cayenne balm, this cooling balm may be used for again ache if you decide you do not much like the warm temperature from the cayenne. It's awesome and sparkling, and it'll help with even excessive pain. Make effective to apply it if you enjoy the start of a few soreness coming without delay to for its maximum gain. The natural restoration houses of Eucalyptus oil will help you in assuaging stiffness, similarly to peppermint and camphor oils.

Ingredients:

1. ½ cup of coconut oil

2. 2 teaspoons of grated beeswax

3. Five-6 drops of Camphor oil

four. Five-6 drops of Peppermint Essential oil

5. Five Drops of Eucalyptus Essential oil

Directions:

1. Using a double boiler, combination collectively the coconut oil and beeswax. Stir it together over a low hearth in order that it mixes together. Make certain to keep stirring so it does not start to burn.

2. Remove from the hearth and upload on your Camphor, Peppermint, and Eucalyptus oils. Pour into your favored bins to permit cool. A tin can or glass jar that you may seal tightly is good. Rub into troubled sore regions on your another time.

#three Balm - Comfrey Cooling Balm

Comfrey leaves are a few specific all herbal difficulty that can useful resource in easing your again pains as an opportunity unexpectedly. It is beneficial for all over again ache, bruises, sprains, further to joint illness. It works on problem spots throughout, so when you mixture this proper into a balm, it's going to provide instant remedy in your achy once more A suitable concept is to add peppermint in your balm as a cooling agent on the way to offer a further prolonged-lasting impact to lower your pain.

Ingredients:

1. 10 drops of Peppermint Essential oil

2. ½ cup of Coconut oil

three. 2 teaspoons of grated Beeswax

4. ¼ cup of dried Comfrey Leaves

Directions:

1. Mix your comfrey leaves and coconut oil together in a medium pot over a low fireplace for about an hour. To avoid burning, stir occasionally after which filter out the leaves.

2. Using a double boiler, blend collectively the beeswax and infused oil. Stir collectively over a low fireside and then combination in the peppermint crucial oil.

3. Remove from the flame and pour into your desired bins to allow cool. A tin can or glass jar that you can seal tightly is good. Rub into sore areas in your again.

#4 Balm- Blended Arnica Balm

The strength of Arnica flowers additionally recognized as an great pain remedy treatment for returned ache. This herbal flower includes houses which may be very powerful for pain, mainly at the same time as you combine it with lavender as a calming agent. Adding peppermint also makes for a pleasant aggregate with a view to relax any flared-up muscles in the decrease lower back. Mix those materials together and word for yourself how an awful lot better you can feel at the same time as you rub them in on your stricken spots

Ingredients:

1. ¼ teaspoon of lavender crucial oil

2. ¼ teaspoon of peppermint important oil

three. ½ cup of beeswax granules

4. 6 oz. Of dried arnica plants

five. 2 cups of coconut oil

Directions:

1. Pour coconut oil into a massive pot for an hour over a low flame. Mix inside the arnica plants and stir frequently to avoid any burning.

After an hour, clean out the final plant life leaving behind the infused coconut oil.

2. Using a double boiler, mixture together the beeswax and infused oil. Stir collectively over a low fireplace and then aggregate in the peppermint and lavender crucial oils.

three. Remove from the flame and pour into your preferred boxes to allow cool. A tin can or glass jar that you may seal tightly is proper. Rub into stricken sore regions in your yet again

#5 Balm - Plantain Balm

A lot of mother and father anticipate that plantain is a weed, however it is also a very beneficial issue for any pain assuaging balm. When implemented topically it is tested to reduce infection. Plantain is likewise ideal for bruises and skin breakouts. Adding a few peppermint oil also can upload a calming gain, at the side of clove oil which may be used as a numbing component, which allows in expediting ache comfort.

Ingredients:

1. 2 teaspoons grated beeswax

2. ½ cup of coconut oil

three. 10 drops of peppermint crucial oil

four. Five drops clove crucial oil

5. ¼ cup of plantain leaves

6. 1 teaspoon of red pepper cayenne powder

Directions:

1. Pour coconut oil into a huge pot and mix inside the purple pepper cayenne and simmer over a low flame for about 2.Five hours stirring often to keep away from any burning.

2. Using a double boiler, mixture together the beeswax and infused oil. Stir together over a low fireside and then mixture inside the critical oils.

3. Remove from the flame and pour into your chosen containers to allow cool. A tin can or glass jar that you may seal tightly is good. Rub into sore areas for your again

Salve #6 Soothing Pain Relief

Oils made from lavender are recognized for its ability to ease soreness within the muscle businesses, and roman chamomile has similar houses too. It's amazing for relaxation and decreasing inflamed muscle groups similarly to the feelings of worry and tension. Feel free to use this aggregate liberally to your strained areas.

Ingredients:

1. ½ cup of coconut oil

2. 10 drops of peppermint crucial oil

3. 2 teaspoons of grated beeswax

4. 10 drops of roman chamomile important oil

five. 15 drops of lavender vital oil

Directions:

1. Using a double boiler, aggregate together the beeswax and coconut oil. Stir together over a low fireside until melted together.

2. Pour for your critical oils till they will be very well combined. Remove from the flame and pour into your preferred packing containers to permit cool. A tin can or glass jar that you can seal tightly is ideal. Rub into troubled sore regions on your once more

Chapter 5: How It Really Works Inside The Fight In Competition To Weight Issues

Since the body desires additional heating in water, it has to dissipate a lot more power than on land.

Taking below consideration that being overweight is usually a direct contraindication to severe physical interest and heavy hundreds, water aerobics will assist those who want to get their figure in order without harming their fitness.

The effect is furnished due to the truth that:

• The massage effect of the water softens the pores and skin, gently solving the hassle.

• Additional electricity is expended inside the water to maintain a strong and strong position inside the water, in addition to to triumph over resistance to water (for assessment, the pushing pressure of water is at the least 12 instances that of air).

• Due to the lack of strong manual below someone's toes, they need to art work plenty harder and be extra energetic.

• An greater fats burning effect is supplied via the usage of the temperature distinction among the temperature of the human body and that of the aquatic environment.

• Exercise is conducive.

• The mental thing furthermore plays an further critical function: the frame of a person inside the water is shape of really hidden from prying eyes. This method that someone is not going to care how it appears from the outdoor. This negates the complexes, giving anyone the possibility to experience more comfortable.

How are the commands

Classes are held in water, the temperature of this is in the variety of 28 to 33 stages. The depth of the pool water can variety. The duration of education for novices does not exceed forty five minutes, the pace is chosen as an opportunity moderate. The most vital issue at this degree is to accustom the body to being in an unusual environment, to place the breath. And moreover study the only, which does now not require particular training actions.

A traditional exercising consists of the following steps:

- To warmth.

- Extension.

- Special physical video games for the development of all muscle organizations.

- Exercises to increase patience, flexibility and power.

- Hitch.

To higher put together for the lesson, in advance than education, you need to warm up nicely on land, getting organized the body for pressure. This will assist the frame to fast get used to the new surroundings and will make the muscle tissues greater elastic. After the lesson, it is endorsed to swim a chunk greater and do at least.

In cutting-edge, an hour of intensive water aerobics schooling permits you to burn at least seven hundred kcal. And ordinary education will offer you with the possibility to miss about the trouble of more weight for a long term.

For novices, the training software consists of the most effective bodily video games. It consists of:

- Swing your legs

- Pulling the legs closer to the chest

- Skip

An superior company can manipulate to pay for an advanced application. Consists in:

- Walking and strolling more extreme.

- Swing your legs (in a single-of-a-type tips).

- Classic.

- Dance health factors.

As the period of the lesson will growth to an hour, the depth of the hundreds will increase. Those who've been engaged in this form of fitness for numerous years can discover the coins for:

- Exercise with weights

Some of the maximum commonplace and effective water aerobics embody:

- To shape the body and reduce the waist.

- The hands are closed at the extent of the solar plexus. The elbows relaxation inside the route of the stomach, in the fingers, overcoming the resistance of the water, they rest within the path of the chest.

- Turning the frame sideways

- Leans in superb suggestions

- To form the hips and stomach:

- Swing your legs up and down

- "Scissors" - pass-legged swings

- Seated armrest

- Slim thighs

- Bend your knees at the same time as pulling inside the path of your chest

- jumping out of the water

- Leg line modeling

- Jump jumps

- Walk and run in the water

How many kg are you able to shed kilos?

Regular exercising allows you to frequently lose as a minimum 6 kilograms in step with month. You can also beautify the effect with the help of giving up terrible conduct, and lots of others.

Advantages and downsides

What are the advantages of a person who first comes to a selection to do water aerobics?

• Exercising within the water places a whole lot much less pressure on the frame.

• In the water, the skeleton and muscle groups are a good deal much less state of affairs to effect and damage because they're no longer stricken by the stress of gravity. In addition, the opposing thrust stress acts at the water, which furthermore helps lessen the burden at the body. In the water, you can combine pretty excessive and complex movements with out a extraordinary deal hazard.

• Water aerobics has a slight effect on the joints, without detrimental, but at the other, heals them and expands their abilities. This makes it appropriate even for the disabled and the elderly.

• The water allows you to carry out physical video video games of this form of diploma of complexity that a person may additionally need to every now and then do them with out unique schooling on land.

• The economic financial savings scheme permits you to seriously boom the period of traditional hobby.

• Water massage reduces the quantity of lactic acid in muscle tissues. This permits you to almost no longer revel in tired neither after training nor tomorrow.

• Classes will let you hone movement precision and electricity.

• Water contributes to the overall hardening of the frame, improves blood go together with the flow, relieves muscle anxiety

• Due to the strengthening of the stabilizing muscle tissue, posture alignment happens.

• With varicose veins, this type of aerobics stimulates the outflow of venous blood, relieves the coronary coronary coronary heart valves and reduces the danger of blood stagnation in today's.

• In humans with excessive blood pressure, there is a decrease on this indicator.

• Separately, it is properly really worth noting the exciting impact, sleep development, ordinary universal overall performance development and mood elevation, it truely is supplied to individuals who determined to function to this uncommon form of pressure.

There are just a few downsides to water aerobics, similarly to contraindications. This form of health is typically advocated for the widest sort of humans, irrespective of health diploma, age, and lots of others.

Contraindications

Thanks to the mild mode, water aerobics are almost unrestricted. However, it's far contraindicated in people with thrombophlebitis. Strengthens muscle corporations, normalizes respiratory, the paintings of the cardiovascular device and has a beneficial impact on fitness.

A new direction in fitness is gaining recognition: water aerobics. What opinions say approximately water aerobics for weight reduction, how effective it's miles, how useful it's miles, the ones and one of a kind questions may be discussed further.

Water aerobics is a exceedingly new health area in which all dance movements and physical activities are achieved within the water. The trainings are determined by means of way of manner of musical accompaniment.

It is the first-rate and most steady gymnastics as compared to unique regions. Water enables the frame, therefore the possibility of harm is minimal. Exercising within the water requires extra strive, which places extra excessive strain on the muscle companies.

In addition, the following elements are used:

In maximum instances, the schooling are held inside the pool, in which the water reaches chest stage. Workouts lasting forty-60 minutes provide the most benefit.

Now permit's discover how frequently each week you want to do water aerobics to shed pounds. As a rule of thumb, three exercises in step with week are enough for those more pounds to steadily start to disappear.

The blessings of water aerobics for weight loss:

• relaxes nerve endings and relieves pressure;

• all muscle companies are worried within the physical sports, incl. Muscular tissues of internal organs;

• trains respiratory resistance;

• has a exceptional effect at the artwork of the cardiovascular gadget;

• normalizes glucose ranges;

• softens the burden at the joints;

• has a awesome impact on the health of pregnant girls;

• create a appropriate temperature regime - the frame does now not overheat;

• dispose of the signs and symptoms;

• makes the pores and skin greater elastic and elastic;

• strain is normalized.

How powerful are aerobics and is an extra set of measures desired?

Having enrolled in aquatic fitness, girls are interested by the question of whether or not or now not water aerobics are useful for weight reduction, whether or no longer or not extra strategies are wanted. It must be cited that the calorie loss in water is lots less than with similar sports sports in nature and through the years on land. But for mild, mild weight loss, aquatic fitness by myself will suffice.

The second no an awful lot less important component: do water aerobics help in the direction of cellulite? A individual overcomes water resistance, stimulates blood movement and strengthens muscle tissues.

It is way to the hydromassage impact that the fats deposits begin to interrupt down. Water is a type of simulator, way to which the muscle agencies attain the vital load, however do no longer get worn-out.

Can I do it myself or do I need an teacher?

Some ladies, after going to more than one education, decide to teach on their very personal. But, will it is in this example the advantage of water aerobics for weight loss, or is it higher to exercise with an teacher? Here are a few reasons to go through in mind instructor-led commands:

For protection motives, it is remarkable not to train by myself. It is critical to hold in thoughts that water is an element, it's far higher to exercise below the supervision of a in a position individual.

Group instructions convey human beings collectively. As a preferred rule, schooling is only below the guidance of an instructor.

The instructor will manual, advise on what and the manner to art work to gain an powerful end cease result.

For humans with injuries, ailments, weight problems, it's far encouraged to conduct education first-rate with an trainer.

Chapter 6: Yoga Tips For Beginners

To begin running toward yoga, you virtually do no longer have to be bendy. As a keep in mind of fact, yoga will help you switch out to be flexible. Since there are lots of severa yoga patterns which variety from slight to complete of life, you could look for yoga teacher and fashion on the way to exceptional fit your dreams, beauty time table, modern physical state of affairs, barriers and skills.

Be sure that your instructor is aware about any fitness problems and your diploma of fitness. Do now not stress any poses or moves. Mastery of yoga poses will consist of everyday exercise. Wear stretchable or gently loose apparel which can be cushty. Expect to take off your shoes in the end of a yoga session.

At the end of a yoga consultation, you have to revel in calm and invigorated and no longer in bodily pain. Try attending yoga lessons for two times consistent with week or maybe extra. A unmarried yoga consultation typically lasts for about 60 minutes.

Following are some hints for yoga beginners:

1. Select a particular yoga kind

This step consists of doing some studies for your element. A lot of yoga instructions are to be had to be had, and you may be most probably to be disappointed in case you pick out out a certain yoga type that does not in shape your country of bodily health and individual.

Take a few minutes to study the evaluation of yoga as furnished at the primary financial wreck of this e-book. For majority of yoga starters, vinyasa or hatha yoga beauty can be the most suitable, relying on whether you would like to transport for a quick or sluggish-paced beauty. Keep in thoughts that these are just clean yoga instructions and you can normally skip for a few element extra advanced or fancier later.

2. Look for a yoga elegance

Try seeking out yoga training to be had in your locality. You also can have a have a look at on-line sources, nearby alternative newspapers further to health and health magazines for listings.

Go for a yoga studio this is reachable on your art work or home in order that it'd be clean in case you need to get into beauty. Be remarkable to start with a vital stage yoga splendor. A lot of health facilities and gyms also offer yoga durations – this is a excellent region to get started in case you are already a gymnasium member. Finding a in a position yoga instructor will assist you to live with your yoga training.

three. Know what to carry during yoga training

During the number one day of your yoga class, you can now not should carry pretty a few stuff besides for your self and some breathable, comfortable clothing. Majority of yoga studious have yoga mats available for condominium.

four. Know what to expect

In a regular yoga beauty, the contributors located their yoga mats in a unfastened grid managing the the front of the room. This is generally identifiable through way of the teacher's mat or a small altar. It is strongly advised now not to line up your yoga mat exactly with one next to it because you and your co-yogi would require a few area in a few yoga regions. The individuals commonly take a seat in a pass-legged characteristic.

The yoga teacher might also moreover begin the beauty by the usage of manner of predominant the splendor in reciting the syllable "om" 3 times. Depending at the instructor, there might be a few quick meditation or some breathing carrying activities at the begin of the session.

This is typically located via heat-up yoga poses, then more whole of existence poses. Next might be stretches and directly to the very last relaxation. If you want a few relaxation at any time, take a toddler's pose.

Oftentimes, the instructor will roam spherical to every participant at some point of the very last relaxation and provide them with a piece massage. Majority of yoga teachers give up the session with some distinct set of "oms".

The Do's and Don'ts in some unspecified time in the future of a Yoga Class

Do's:

• Familiarize yourself with some of starter's yoga poses earlier than taking your first yoga session

• Ask the yoga trainer for assist if you want it

• Inform your yoga teacher that it's going to be your first yoga session

• Review yoga etiquette so that you will feel very comfortable in a very surprising state of affairs

• Come decrease decrease again in multiple days on your next yoga session

Don'ts:

• Wear socks or shoes at some point of yoga periods

• Drink water in the course of the session, notwithstanding the fact that have some in advance than and after the beauty

• Have an extraordinary meal right earlier than a yoga consultation. Try to eat slight more than one hours in advance than the session begins offevolved

Chapter 7: Bodyweight Exercises For The Chest/Back, Shoulders/Arms And Core!

Now that the total body and leg muscle groups had been taken care of, allow's observe some of the opportunity components of your body. For an entire and beneficial exercising consultation, reputation on all additives or muscle organizations of the body. Include a few physical sports from every class to make sure that all your muscle businesses are in addition toned and bolstered in a manner that ensures a whole body increase, development and fitness.

Chest and Back Exercises:

Standard Push-Up: This is simply a traditional and works every unmarried time in flexing the muscles of the chest and yet again respectively. Stand to your ft collectively collectively along with your arms apart at shoulder width and make certain that your feet live flexed at the space of a hip. Tighten your center muscle agencies and start bending the elbows until your chest reached close to the ground after which push your self up yet again. While doing this exercise guarantees that your elbows live intently tucked for your body.

85

Dolphin Push Up: Place your self at a dolphin characteristic, it is in conjunction with your elbows at the floor. Start thru leaning earlier and grade by grade lowering your shoulders until your head remains over your hands. Now, pull your fingers up and bypass returned to the start function. Repeat the step some times.

Donkey Kick: Now is the time to get things going critical. Place your self in a push up characteristic, even as keeping your legs together. Kick your legs into the air, while making sure that your middle muscular tissues continue to be engaged, knees remain bent and goal the toes backwards in the course of the glutes. Once accomplished, land lightly and soar another time to the beginning characteristic and repeat.

Superman: Always desired some incredible powers? Try this exercise and your frame may be at its bendy notable. Place yourself down on the ground in conjunction with your face going thru the floor. Extend your legs and arms respectively. Keep your lower back or torso however and try lifting your legs and arms concurrently. Your frame ought to form a small curve which makes your muscular tissues tighten efficiently. Repeat some instances and your chest and back muscle groups can be more potent with time and exercising.

Headstand Push Up: This circulate is outstanding ideal for the experts or the expert obtainable who can circulate their body like a miracle. For novices, it's far first rate advocated to get the help or help of a pal or a companion to complete this instead beneficial exercise. Start thru getting yourself on a head stand characteristic along side your head at the floor and your legs excessive up towards the wall. Prop yourself on your elbows at an attitude of 90 degrees and attempt a pushup which is the alternative way up. Your head need to go with the flow up and down whilst your legs remain intact in its function.

Reverse Fly: upward push up tall along with your frame in a proper away function. Extend one leg beforehand and bend the knees barely. Engage the abs muscle tissues and gently bend earlier from the waist with fingers prolonged inside the route of the edges. Ensure that your shoulder blades continue to be squeezed through out. Repeat the steps a few instances.

Shoulders and Arms Exercise:

Triceps Dip: Place yourself down on the ground close to an increased surface. With your knees slightly bent, take hold of the corner of the heightened ground and straighten out your arms. Bend your hands to an angle of ninety levels and straighten it all over again at the identical time as your heels stay driven within the course of the floor. To growth the intensity of the exercise, increase the proper hand whilst attractive the left leg as opposites provide extra challenge.

Boxer: begin thru retaining your ft aside at the width of a hip. Keep your knees bent and your elbows tucked in and at the equal time as doing this extend one arm in advance and the alternative backward. Once you revel in the pull, deliver your palms collectively and try once more thru switching hands respectively. Repeat it a few instances and you could truly get no longer truly your muscle groups however also your boxing actions proper on fletch!

Arm Circles: This is a easy reduce way to get your shoulder blades and palms flex for excessive electricity and strength. Stand at the aspect of your palms extended out toward your sides in a manner that they stay perpendicular to the location of the torso. Star making small circles along aspect your arms, first in a clockwise characteristic and preserve it for a few seconds and then anti clock clever. Repeat some instances will you revel in the muscle companies tightening.

Core Exercises:

L Seat: Seat yourself without problems at the floor and extend your legs in a way that your ft remain flexed. Begin with the useful resource of slightly rounding your torso together together with your arms located on the ground and often bring your hips, keep for some seconds and lighten up. Repeat and loosen up some times. This workout works wonders in strengthening your center muscle corporations which in flip ends in expanded energy, power and a in shape body.

Flutter Kick: Lie down at the ground, putting your palms on the rims and our arms going thru the ground. Start via extending your legs and gradually decorate your ft from the ground approximately 6 to 7 inches. Try to make tiny up and down actions along with your legs at the same time as making sure that the center muscle tissue continue to be engaged thru out.

Side plank: Roll over on your thing and try to prop your self up on one elbow and foot respectively. Gradually get your middle muscle groups engaged and lift your hips and gold them tight for a few seconds to a minute or perhaps longer. Hold on for so long as u can for wonderful effects. This is one of the nice strategies of provide a boost in your center tremendously.

Russian Twist: Seat yourself at the floor together with your feet collectively and knees barely bent. Lift your toes a few inches from the ground and float your fingers slowly from one side to the opportunity creating a twisting movement. Try to take it sluggish because of the reality this is at the same time as your muscle tissues will flex and tighten the maximum. The slower the twist, the better the pull you may feel.

Bicycle: This one within reason easy and can be completed via anyone. Lie down to your decrease again along with your knees bent and maintain your hands under your head. Lift your head barely and convey your proper knee closer to the chest while extending your left elbow in the path of it. Keep alternating the legs and the elbows and opposites guarantees most engagement of the middle muscular tissues. Keep cycling with the useful resource of appealing your knees and elbows in the long run.

Crunch: Lie down flat at the floor and make sure that your knees stay bent and your ft contact the floor flat. Place your arms beneath your hair and reduce your chin a bit. Now, grade by grade try to improve yourself off your again and curl your frame within the route of the toes. Lift your self simply halfway till you sense your middle tighten and engage itself completely. Once curled, maintain your self notwithstanding the truth that for some seconds, retreat to the begin and repeat some times.

Abdominal Press: Yet a few distinct effective exercise plan to get the middle going robust. Lie down on the ground at the side of your ft pressed to the floor. Bend your knees barely and tighten the middle. Gradually, increase your proper leg collectively along with your knees and hip bent to an perspective of ninety degree. Extend your right hand earlier to touch the lifted knee. As you attain in advance, you could experience your muscle tissues tighten considerably. Stay on the modern characteristic for a few seconds and cross again t your starting characteristic. Now, attempt once more with the opportunity leg. Keep repeating the exercise, even as switching or alternating legs and palms respectively.

Chapter 8: The Psychology Of Change

for maximum people, the phrase trade manner PAIN. No one wants to go through the pain of exchange.

Even while we are in pain and suffering, sometimes it's a great deal less complicated to stay that manner than it is to trade. So how are we able to get beyond the pain of trade?

The super element we are able to do is discover the energy of the Psychology of Change— the energy of the notable attitude.

The Psychology of Change states that you may be maximum a fulfillment in developing new behavior thru the use of adding small, beneficial steps first.

The worst difficulty you may do is test your lifestyles and say, "Oh my gosh, I'm no longer transferring as an awful lot as I ought to. I need to head be a part of a health club and do a three-month intensive utility so I can workout all day, each day!"

I've seen multiple failures in the enthusiastic beginner's mindset. Such overzealous wondering crashes speedy.

Now, in case you are inspired to make a dramatic way of life trade, by way of manner of the use of all technique move for it!

If you sense like you have got the sources, guide device, and past successes, then, thru using all method pass for it!

For the relaxation people, we can must depend upon what the Psychology of Change teaches us. We will want to define the subsequent step.

According to the Psychology of Change, humans may have the most achievement in the event that they start small—taking toddler steps.

You can start including more motion on your life with the useful aid of:

• going for a stroll greater often

• extending the period of your stroll

• placing your alarm ten minutes earlier to stand up and carry out a little very simple variety-of-motion carrying sports activities

- including more than one yoga poses or more than one stretches on your morning ordinary

Start small however take intentional steps to characteristic more movement into your day.

This technique works because of the reality we have a propensity to assemble momentum as we begin which include and accumulating small successes.

We see ourselves converting with out a ache!

You set the guidelines.

Take motion at the quantity you agree with will give you the outcomes you need.

My desire is that no matter in that you are on the pastime spectrum, your next infant step may be this one clean exercise for posture—the foundation of motion.

Start with baby steps.

The Y-T-W-L

T

he Y-T-W-L is an workout seemed within the health enterprise for being a part of a shoulder exercise circuit.

Normally, you lay face down on an incline bench and use weights to construct shoulder electricity along side your hands in unique positions.

The exercising that I'm recommending is changed to be finished as a standing postural stretch an awesome way to rock your international!

You will now not need weights or an incline bench. You exceptional want your frame and your palms!

I ought to offer credit score score where credit rating is due. This exercise as a postural stretch comes from actually one in every of my mentors inside the chiropractic, fitness and fitness realm, Dr. James Chestnut.

The letters represent the posture positions inside the workout, however Dr. Chestnut additionally came up with high-quality imagery to in form the acronym.

Y-T-W-L stands for Youthful-Thoughtful-Wise-Loving.

Dr. Chestnut is the developer and lead teacher of the Post-Graduate Wellness Lifestyle

Certification software for the International Chiropractors Association. He is developing a huge amount of exchange within the international.

He has stimulated hundreds of chiropractors to live a more fit manner of existence themselves and train their sufferers on the way to achieve this as well.

He has been at the leading edge of manner of life health.

Let's walk thru this exercising step-with the resource of-step.

Each letter represents a characteristic your hands are going to be in. So, you guessed it; it's type of just like the loopy Y-M-C-A dance track.

For every arm function (letter), you could have the same stance. You can do the Y-T-W-L sitting; but, it's miles going to be greater powerful if you're status.

Let's get commenced out. It is beneficial to try this exercising in the the front of a reflect. Then, you can make sure that you have appropriate form.

First, allow's get into the right status role. Ready?

The Stance:

• Stand collectively collectively with your toes shoulder-width aside.

• Engage your center muscle mass by means of the usage of bracing your abs like someone is going to punch you within the stomach. Tighten your muscle companies on your lower lower decrease back. But now not too tight. Make fine you may despite the fact that breathe.

• Put your shoulders down and reduce back so it looks as if you are trying to deliver your shoulder blades near together. Imagine attempting to drag your shoulder blades down and again, like you are tucking them into your another time pockets of your pants or shorts.

By absolutely standing in this feature, you could experience hundreds of hysteria already and that's k!

Work on keeping the proper stance feature some times an afternoon and stretch those postural muscle groups!

When you're beginning to revel in a terrific deal much less tension at the same time as you stand that way, go with the flow directly to the arm positions.

The Y

• In the correct stance, hold your fingers up over your head.

• Point your thumbs straight away inside the returned of you.

• Get your hands as right away as possible, with little to no bend in your elbows (if you can).

• Start through retaining that role for five-10 seconds and work up to fifteen-30 seconds.

That is the Youthful function.

The T

• As you preserve your thumbs pointing behind you, permit your hands to drop horizontal with the floor.

• Again, get your arms as proper now as feasible, eliminating the bend within the elbows as a bargain as you could.

• Start thru shielding that position for five-10 seconds and art work up to fifteen-30 seconds.

That is the Thoughtful function.

The W

From the T characteristic:

• Drop your elbows down toward the ground.

• Your thumbs ought to however point within the returned of you.

• Check in to make certain you're nonetheless retaining the perfect stance together with your shoulders down and lower back and your shoulder blades drawn collectively in the direction of the backbone.

• Start with the aid of way of maintaining that characteristic for 5-10 seconds and paintings up to fifteen-30 seconds.

You are really in the Wise role.

The L

• From the Wise function, bring your elbows into the sides of your body like you are making a ninety-diploma mindset collectively along side your hands.

• Point your thumbs right now in the again of you.

• Start with the aid of preserving that function for five-10 seconds and artwork up to fifteen-30 seconds.

That is the Loving feature.

To see my instructional video demonstrating the Y-T-W-L exercise, visit: www.Theelevationprinciple.Com/ytwl/.

Do this workout as a minimum times a day.

An smooth time to do this is first problem even as you upward push up within the morning. Maybe in advance than you get inside the shower. And as an opportunity proper earlier than you go to bed.

You will have even greater achievement with this if you do that during the day, preferably 1-2 extra instances in some unspecified time in the future of the day.

Work as a incredible deal as protecting every arm position for at least 15 seconds. The extra you're able to complete this exercise finally of the day, the a bargain a great deal less time you need to take with every arm characteristic.

This is designed to be a lifestyle exercising, due to this it becomes a part of your every day dependancy, just like brushing your enamel.

This postural stretch workout is designed to counteract the consequences of sitting and neck strain related to ahead head posture because of generation use.

Sugar is to enamel what sitting is to the backbone.

The Time to Change is Now

A

s a populace, you can now go searching and resultseasily discover that 60%-ninety% of the people you word at paintings, in airports, department stores or anywhere in public have their heads buried in an digital device.

Forward head posture is an epidemic within the making. We frequently supply our 2-year-olds digital devices to maintain them occupied and entertained. Even if toddlers are using devices for "academic" purposes, we're letting them interact in an hobby this is wreaking havoc on how their neck will feature. It will negatively have an effect on their health.

But you may do some thing superb approximately it for your self, your family, your friends, and your co-employees.

You can counteract ahead head posture and cast off your neck pain, as quickly as and for all!

Do the Y-T-W-L exercise and over the years you may examine that now not only does your neck function better and float better, you can enjoy better too.

You will rise up straighter.

Your shoulders will rest down and decrease again.

You will lose lots of anxiety for your higher once more and neck, and your chin can be held up high.

Tension headaches will dissipate.

Jaw tension will loosen up.

You'll breathe deeper and sleep better.

Your self notion will increase, too.

Did that, subconsciously, our posture affects our ordinary revel in of properly-being?

You've seen it. When you word your buddies in a frustrated, depressed u . S . A ., they typically look down loads. They have a have a observe the floor, and their shoulders are rounded ahead.

The Y-T-W-L workout can assist them actually contrary that. It is viable to alternate an emotional nation by way of converting posture!

Choose to gain this.

The Y-T-W-L is a easy exercising that you could do as a minimum times an afternoon and upwards of three-4 instances an afternoon, especially if you take a seat masses.

I have been in chiropractic exercise for extra than 12 years and I actually have witnessed extremely good fulfillment with this exercising.

We have seen humans that have come into the office with three-four inches of forward head posture. This exercise, on the aspect of receiving chiropractic changes, has allowed them to effect unconscious muscle memory patterns and create the change had to help their lifestyle.

We pay attention people say, "I try to rise up at once," or, "I try to be extra privy to it and capture myself more frequently."

That is terrific to be more aware of your posture, however the backside line is, your posture and how your body holds itself is really subconscious.

It is like telling a child to sit up straight in elegance. They most effective collect this as long as their hobby is focused on sitting up right away. Once their interest is going somewhere else, they are going to move lower returned to slouching once more.

The Y-T-W-L workout will art work those subconscious muscle reminiscence styles to counteract the ahead head posture and create new, stronger, more strong patterns.

Chapter 9: Standing Yoga Poses

Having accurate balance is lots more than the capability to face properly on one foot. While that is a terrific feat to collect with yoga, right balance encompasses your physical, mental, and emotional balance. Standing yoga poses will help you've got were given better attention, triumph over stress, address difficult situations extra lightly, and most significantly, undergo lifestyles with more calm and attention.

Here are status yoga poses you can start with:

1: The Standing Mountain Pose (Tadasana)

Benefits

• Improves stability

• Builds posture

• Enhances attention

• Opens up your chest hole area for respiratory wearing activities

• Stimulates thyroid and allows increase your height.

Instructions

Stand erect together with your ft saved together and your fingers placed at your sides. Keep your weight lightly unfold and pressed in the path of the arches and balls of your toes. Breathe in rhythmically and grade by grade. If attaining stability is hard, step your feet about 6 inches aside or wider.

Keep your legs straightened out, and draw down thru the heels with the toes grounded firmly into the earth. Then draw the topmost a part of the thighs up after which lower once more.

Slightly tuck your tailbone with out rounding your lower decrease once more. Extend through your torso. Free your shoulder blades from your head in the direction of the lowest of your waist.

Enlarge in the course of your collarbones together with your shoulders stored in keeping with the sides of your body.

Keep your shoulder blades corporation within the direction of your decrease back ribs without squeezing them collectively. Maintain proper away fingers, expand your palms downwards, and keep your triceps enterprise organization.

Extend your neck whilst maintaining your breathe even and smooth. Gently gaze at the horizon. Hold this pose for approximately 60 seconds, and then lighten up your complete body.

2: The Chair Pose (Utkatasana)

Benefits

• Improves your posture

• Tones your leg muscular tissues excellently

• Enhances your balance

• Tones your thighs and abdomen

• Great for runners and one-of-a-type athletes

• Stimulates the organs, your coronary coronary heart, diaphragm, and abdomen

Instructions

Start within the mountain pose and keep your feet together collectively together along with your big feet touching; if that is too hard to do, step your feet apart about a hip-distance.

Inhale deeply at the same time as raising your arms above your head and make sure the fingers are perpendicular to the floor.

Exhale and bend your knees at the same time as bringing your thighs as parallel to the floor as they may be capable of get. Your knees need to protrude barely over your feet and your torso should shape an proper right mind-set over your thighs. Make great you shift your weight into your heels.

Slightly tilt your head backwards as you gaze progressively at a factor among your fingers.

Hold for approximately 60 seconds after which breathe in deeply and straighten your legs at the same time as you increase through your fingers. Finally, exhale and release returned to your location to start, the Mountain Pose.

three: The Pyramid Pose (Parsvottanasana)

We furthermore name this fame pose the Intense Side Stretch.

Benefits

• Stretches your spines, hips, hamstrings, and shoulders

• Improves your stability and posture

• Helps calm your thoughts

- Cools the mind and soothes the concerned gadget

- Tones the liver and the spleen

Instructions

Start within the Mountain Pose. Turn on your left and maintain your ft 2-three toes aside. Keep your palms firmly located for your hips. Align your hips, after which turn your proper the the front foot approximately 90 degrees to maintain its ft pointing to the top of your yoga mat. Also, turn your left returned foot about 60 tiers to keep the ft pointing in the route of the pinnacle of your yoga mat. Then turn to ensure you're going through the course of your the front foot.

Draw your left feet a chunk bit ahead and rectangular your hips to the top of your mat.

Reach your hands out closer to your factors after which draw them in the back of your back at the same time as keeping your elbows clasped. Alternatively, you may convey the arms right proper right into a opposite prayer function clearly in the returned of your again with the arms urgent together at the same time as you attain the hands within the direction of the pinnacle.

Extend the torso on the identical time as you are breathing in. As you exhale, make certain to fold the hips then extend the torso over the the front legs. Ensure you preserve the duration of the backbone. Ensure the crown of the top extends beforehand together with your tailbone accomplishing in the back of you.

Ground your self down thru the heel of your back foot whilst watching on the huge toe of your the the the front foot.

Hold this pose for about 60 seconds. Press firmly thru your decrease back heel and barely supply your torso to release yourself from this pose. Release each arms and preserve your palms in your hips. Change the place of your ft and repeat the gadget on the opposite aspect.

4: The Tree Pose (Vrksasana)

Benefits

• Helps assemble self-self guarantee and vanity

• Helps to procure pelvic stability

• Helps stretch your thighs

- Improves your stability

- Strengthens your hips, shoulders and torso

- Builds strength at your calves, ankles and has healing effects on flat feet

Instructions

Start in the Mountain pose. Shift your weight on your left foot. Keep your right knee bent, after which obtain down and keep your right ankle in a commercial enterprise enterprise grip. Use your hand to draw the proper foot alongside the inner left thigh. Ensure that you don't relaxation the foot towards the knee. You can quality rest your foot above or underneath your knee. If accomplishing stability is tough, preserve the simplest of your right foot located along your internal ankle even as resting your feet on the ground.

Bring the arms to relaxation at the hips and then proceed to growth the tailbone in the direction of the ground. Keep your proper foot pressed firmly into the left thigh.

Ensure both arms are lightly resting at the hips. You can enlarge your fingers above your head carrying out your fingertips inside the direction of the sky for extra task after which turn up your head to gaze between the two raised hands.

Hold this pose for approximately 60 seconds, step your toes together another time, and repeat the method on the other factor.

5: Triangle Pose (Utthita Trikonasana)

Benefits

• Fosters weight reduction and tones waist

• Helps you purchased stability

• Stretches your groin and inner thighs

• Improves digestion

• Increases every bodily and intellectual equilibrium

• Reduces anxiety, again pain, sciatica, and stress

Instructions

Inhale deeply, exhale, and straighten your legs to return right into a triangle pose. You can maintain your proper hand to your ankle, shin, or a block positioned to the out of doors of your proper hand.

Extend your left arm right away over your head

Focus your mind on stacking your left hip over your right hip and your left shoulder over your proper shoulder.

Twist yourself in the route of the ceiling to assist open your chest.

6: Half Moon Pose (Ardha Chandrasana)

Benefits

• Aids strain alleviation

• Improves coordination and stability

• Aids weight reduction

• Helps stretch your ankles and thighs

• Increases intellectual reputation

• Improves digestion

Instructions

Bring your left hand in the path of your left hip. Soften your proper ankle with the aid of way of bending it barely

Keep sliding your right hand beforehand till it's miles about 12-18 inches in the front of your right foot and approximately 6 inches in your proper. You can vicinity a block beneath your hand if you so want.

Lift up your left leg and location it parallel to the floor to help you come into the 1/2-moon pose.

Make positive your left shoulder is right now above your right hand.

Straighten your left arm closer to the ceiling and bring your gaze up on your left hand.

7: Warrior I (Virabhadrasana 1)

Benefits

• Encourages right circulate and breathing

• Energizes your whole body

• Helps shape your hips and calves

• Relaxes your fingers and returned

• Helps make stronger and stretch your thighs and ankles

Instructions

Spin at the ball of your left foot as you drop your left heel proper down to the mat. Your foot should be at an mindset of forty five degrees.

As you inhale, boost up your palms into the Warrior 1 Pose. Ensure each hips are going through the the front of the yoga mat. If you discover this tough t execute, attempt to widen your stance with the aid of the use of slightly shifting each foot in the course of the side edges of the yoga mat.

Extend your the the front knee to carry your proper thigh inside the path of being parallel to the ground.

eight: Warrior II (Virabhadrasana II)

Benefits

• Helps open up your hips

• Stimulates your reproductive organs

• Sharpens your reminiscence

• Stretches and strengthens your calves, ankles, and thighs.

• Improves movement and respiration

• Helps relieve back ache

• Builds stamina and interest

• Therapy for flat toes, osteoporosis, and infertility

Instructions

As you inhale and exhale, open up your hands in order that they're parallel to the floor. As you do this, pull lower back your left hip to preserve you into Warrior 11.

Take a second to take note of the difference among your hip function in Warrior 11 and that of Warrior 1. Your hips are genuinely going thru the left issue of your yoga mat in place of going thru the the front of your mat. Ensure your hips are in a diploma characteristic.

Keep the right knee bent deeply. Pay interest to see if the right knee movements towards the midline then push it once more over the ankle.

nine: Big Toe Pose (Padangusthasana)

Benefits

• Helps you beat strain, anxiety, and moderate melancholy

• Helps relieve insomnia

• Stimulates your kidney and liver

Instructions

Stand right now collectively together with your internal feet parallel and 6 inches aside.

Exhale and bend beforehand out of your hip joints.

Then slide your index and middle palms among your huge and second feet, curl your palms, and firmly grip your ft.

As you inhale, boost your torso as in case you want to rise up again strengthening your elbows.

Lengthen your front torso and alongside side your subsequent inhale, supply your sitting bones, and then decorate the top of your sternum as immoderate as viable. Keep taking deep breaths; boost your torso and agreement your the the front thigh as you attain this and in the end, exhale as you bend your elbows out to the rims

Hold the final characteristic for approximately minute, release your toes, deliver your fingers in your hips, and re-growth your the front torso. With one inhale, swing your head and torso once more to upright as a single unit.

Chapter 10: Strengthening Balance

"Undisturbed calmness of thoughts is attained with the useful resource of cultivating friendliness within the course of the happy, compassion for the sad, pleasure within the virtuous, and indifference towards the wicked."

~ Patañjali

Balance of mind isn't always the simplest form of balance that you purchased from yoga. You also allow yourself to have a look at terrific stability of the body and this is highly vital to power and to slimming down areas of the body which could have out of place their energy thru lazy posture. We get lazy because of the truth the area that we live in nowadays offers a lazy form of lifestyles but that doesn't help you on the same time as you need to be slimmer and keep your body looking appealing and perfectly in trim. However, there are poses that will help you to collect this. The following poses paintings on stability but furthermore they aim particular regions of the body and can help you slim down those regions. The first one offers together with your legs and this embody your higher leg location that could have end up flabby.

The Tree Pose

This pose allows you to stability on one foot however it does a good buy extra than that. The concept of the pose is to help your attention tiers and to reinforce the legs. The tree pose starts offevolved even as you stand for your mat together collectively together with your feet collectively flat at the mat. Your palms start with the beneficial resource of your sides.

Now area your palms into the prayer function in the front of you and raise them in order that the palms of your hands are collectively above your head. It is extraordinarily critical that you hold your once more instantly normally. Lift your left leg and tuck the foot into the internal thigh, at the equal time as retaining your stability perfectly posed. Hold this feature for some moments. Then exhale and allow your foot once more onto the ground, repeating the identical workout with the alternative foot. When your foot is tucked in, your knee want to face outward.

You resemble a tree and also you want to believe the tree status proud within the path of the sky, business organization in its roots and capable of stand without swaying. Do this numerous instances to reinforce your legs. It's honestly proper for balance and your leg strength.

The Chakrasana Pose

This pose enables you with stability as properly however it moreover permits to drag in the ones tummy muscle groups and supply a lift in your arms. It's important which you use a mat, in order that in case you fall, you could no longer injure your self. The mat moreover acts as a first rate floor on your palms and ft and allows them to grip efficaciously in order that the location may be perfected.

This function starts offevolved offevolved via lying on your once more at the mat. It's pretty a comfortable function to start off with as you bend your knees and pull your feet closer on your frame, placing them flat onto the mat. They must be approximately shoulder width apart as they will be going to paintings together with your arms to stability the whole frame.

Thus, having them in the proper feature is critical. The ft ought to be clearly flat always.

Your fingers are then positioned at the element of the pinnacle and the fingertips pointed towards your number one frame. When you bring, you will in fact use the ones to maintain you so that they must be located as flat as viable into the mat with out strain.

On your next inhalation, pick out your frame up so you have it as an extended manner up as possible and your backbone is without a doubt in a bent function. Hold it there. Breathe outside and inside for 1/2 of a dozen instances after which as you exhale the final time, permit your frame back down onto the mat.

This is a brilliant workout for all your frame because it strengthens legs and arms and helps you to experience that tremendous experience of balance and control. If you can't grasp this for your non-public, get a friend that will help you by using manner of placing a hand below your body and helping to useful resource your frame as you increase. This exercising will help your decrease lower back to stay proper now, so subsequently help posture. It may even help you drastically with arm energy and leg energy so that you may be capable of boom the amount of poses that you are capable of do. Remember, you need to in no way pressure sporting sports. Yoga isn't about struggling. It's approximately control and subject. Never forget about this and if you find an exercise is tough to do, attempt another that is inside your capability.

If you do locate this feature difficult, you can moreover advantage from instructions wherein a trainer may be in a function to inform you in which vulnerable point is taking place because of the stance that you are taking. Perhaps a clean movement of your feet role or your hand function will will let you create a super Chakrasana pose. As the word implies, this works to your chakras and permits the float of power through your body.

Chapter 11: Breathing Tips When Running

Proper breathing can be very vital close to taking walks. As going for walks makes use of up pretty a few strength it honestly is derived from burning calories it wishes a number of oxygen for the oxidation of the frame's glucose. Proper breathing can beautify the fatigue resistance of a runner plus their staying strength diploma.

It is generally said that one shouldn't breathe thru the mouth however this isn't genuine as one needs an entire lot of oxygen which cannot be furnished via absolutely the nose. Therefore one want to allow air to go into through the mouth and nose. It is very important which you breathe from the diaphragm or stomach and now not out of your chest. Chest respiratory is pretty shallow and does not allow consumption of enough air unlike deep stomach respiration. This can be very crucial in stopping side stitches that may incapacitate some runners. Exhalation ought to be performed thru the mouth and must be finished definitely in an effort to eliminate all of the carbon dioxide from the lungs and to allow for deep inhalation.

It also can be useful to take three strides on every occasion you inhale and to breathe out every steps. If you have a propensity to be at a pace in which you can't breathe well you then ought to slow down and loosen up and get the time you want to regain your breath lower lower again. It is likewise crucial for novices to take topics slowly as their frame adapts to the situations. Thus, one need to run at a comfortable tempo (conversational pace) in the beginning. The first-rate manner to understand this is to test to peer if you could effects carry out a conversation at the same time as on foot (the communicate take a look at). Remember that questioning an excessive amount of about those tips while jogging can also additionally act in your downside.

Running and Weight Loss

Running is one of the most not unusual methods of losing weight healthily. This is because of the reality it's far pretty exerting on the frame and burns up masses of power which consequently ends in weight loss. A smooth run can dissipate to a hundred calories normal with mile depending on the form of taking walks worried. Running is likewise used as a way of retaining a positive frame form and weight. Apart from going for walks a person looking for to shed pounds have to also keep in thoughts healthy consuming behavior and a healthy life-style with a view to have the pleasant effects.

Runners should have a look at a wholesome eating diet plan because the concept that a runner can consume a few aspect they want as they will burn off the energy is bogus. One need to consequently watch the potions they eat and refrain from overeating. It is usually endorsed to keep home a 'pup bag' even as ingesting out as the quantity of food served in resorts is commonly massive.

The first step to dropping weight is healthful consuming. This is because of the reality you may be capable of superb lose a few pounds in the event that they obtain burning extra strength than they take in. Remember that to lose 1 pound one need to burn 3500 energy. So combining walking with a wholesome diet plan is the fantastic method. The high-quality way to make certain which you do now not overeat at the same time as despite the fact that having the strength needed to run is to conform with a strict diet that specializes in all the meals agencies. Make superb you take smaller portions of food that is immoderate in correct fat and calories and consume a number of entire grains, fruits and greens. Make excessive exceptional to eat until you're nearly full after which prevent to be able to maintain your portions smaller. Do no longer make the error of overcompensating for the strength you burn even as strolling with the aid of taking lots of high calorie beverages and meals as this might bring about weight advantage in choice to loss. This explains why some human beings will be predisposed to gain weight or stay on the identical weight despite taking walks ordinary.

One of the techniques of making sure which you reduce your food consumption is to consume slowly and dispose of any distractions while ingesting. Chewing your meals minimizes risk of overeating as you get to evaluate how your stomach feels. Therefore, you may save you yourself while you feel whole or nearly complete. Distractions which includes searching the television or going for walks on the pc on the same time as consuming growth opportunities of overeating as one is not taking note of their body. Try serving yourself smaller quantities of food or using smaller plates. This assures that you do now not overeat as putting a whole lot of food to your plate consequences in overeating honestly due to the fact it's miles within the the front of you. Another fantastic tip is to begin through manner of taking some stop result and veggies maybe inside the form of salads. This allows fill you up and you switch out to be eating lots much less. As those meals are low in energy you lessen your calorie intake even as not having to go hungry.

It may also additionally additionally help to keep song of what you devour and the amount of energy you eat at every meal. Write the entirety down in a magazine for more than one weeks and this can assist you take a look at suited ingesting behavior. It can even help you see what you might usually tend to brush aside or what you might be overindulging in. This way you could comprehend the quantity of power you want and what's missing from your eating regimen. A journal additionally lets in preserve you disciplined as it serves as a reminder of what to eat or not to eat.

It is likewise very essential to paste to a education agenda. This will assist hold you impacted and could make sure which you burn electricity each day and enhance on your walking. It keeps you prepared and makes positive that you understand what is deliberate for every day. A time desk additionally lets in lessen the possibility of a strolling harm as you will be inclined to do pleasant what you're able and not tackle an excessive amount of too rapid. To provide you with a wonderful time table seek advice from a expert or actually perform a bit studies to discover what works high-quality for you.

If you are not a time table form of person then you definately really definately would probable just favor to do subjects to your personal time. Despite this, it's far very crucial to run frequently if you want to have a few form of consistency that lets in you to shed kilos. Try setting some time aside to run at the least three or 4 instances consistent with week if no longer ordinary. Remember that you can't shed kilos via walking as soon as consistent with week. If you appear to lack the incentive to get out of the residence and run attempt pairing up with someone who can inspire you and keep you business enterprise as you run.

After someday of doing the equal topics over and over once more it gets dull for this reason it's miles essential to hold matters tough. This is great finished with the resource of adding some new techniques and mixing them up collectively together together with your ordinary. Working on your tempo or interval training lets in keep matters glowing. These techniques are quite annoying and dissipate more strength in a shorter term. Speed art work and uphill jogging boom the muscle tissue and enhance the metabolism therefore you burn more power even while you are not running out. Do no longer pressure yourself or overdo these strategies as this will bring about accidents.

Although you have to lessen your calorie intake one must no longer starve or beneath eat. As in advance stated on foot is a traumatic sport so the frame needs sufficient strength so you can carry out this interest. Therefore, skipping food is not actual for a runner because it does not offer your muscle groups sufficient fuel for on foot. A runner want to make certain they devour a balanced food plan and absorb enough calories earlier than, during and even after their session. It is recommended that one take a immoderate calorie food straight away after going for walks as a way to repair the energy used up.

Other Benefits of Running

Apart from loss of weight walking has numerous fitness advantages. These range from the coronary coronary heart to the muscle hobby. Some of the fitness advantages are;

1) Heart: on foot improves arterial elasticity, lowers blood pressure and normally improves the coronary coronary heart's fitness. This reduces risk of a coronary coronary coronary heart attack.

2) Immune device: runners have stronger immune device which reduces threat of infections and contacting illnesses like colds, allergic reactions, menstrual cramps and digestion troubles.

3) Lungs: walking strengthens the lungs and improves lung capability for this reason improves respiration. This is especially outstanding for human beings with a few respiration troubles or the ones who've trouble respiratory. If you have got bronchial asthma, bronchitis or any excessive breathing issues

then one want to be careful at the same time as on foot.

4) Stress reliever: like each exceptional sport, strolling is a pressure reliever. Endorphins released have a tendency to make the man or woman happier usually called a runner's excessive this is powerful in curbing despair. It is idea to boom capability to address every day issues, humor, staying strength and ambition.

5) Circulation: on foot improves the move of blood therefore the tissues get enough supply of vitamins and oxygen and take away waste products. This reduces threat of varicose veins and unique illnesses. Due to superior movement, walking improves brain hobby and complexion by way of technique of creating the pores and pores and skin easy and 'sparkling.'

6) Cancer: research have installed that walking for at least half-hour each day substantially reduces threat of numerous kinds of maximum cancers which includes uterine, breast and gut maximum cancers.

7) Bone density: going for walks will boom bone density specially to your back, legs and hips. It additionally strengthens the muscle

mass and tones them. This reduces hazard of osteoporosis.

eight)   Appetite: taking walks improves one's urge for food as it makes one hungry. This is because it burns power and improves digestion.

nine)   Diabetes: taking walks for at least half-hour every day reduces possibilities of type 2 diabetes.

Running additionally improves mental functioning, boosts self confidence, reduces tension and improves ones moods, as nicely permits with insomnia. Other aerobic bodily activities together with swimming, biking or on foot are nicely for the body.

Common Running Injuries

Although complete of advantages, strolling like every different sport or physical activity consists of a threat of body injuries. This is actual in particular for the vicinity beneath strain, that is, the knee, foot, calf muscle and distinct tendons. Some of the maximum common taking walks accidents are pain related or pulled muscular tissues and tendons. Most of those accidents give up cease result from horrible running method or use of wrong strolling device or over exertion from too much jogging. Therefore, as a runner you should be acquainted with those injuries and recognize a manner to cope with them or maybe in case you must maintain walking or stop it, till restoration.

Pain:

Running can be related to some of muscle pain specifically in the beginning. This in particular impacts the muscle agencies in use which incorporates the calf muscle organizations. In the start the pain can persist for some days (counting on how fit your needs are) and then disappear. It may be treated by using massaging the place and utilizing some warmth at the muscle mass to lighten up them. Pain moreover can be a signal which you are pushing your body an excessive amount of or is probably a signal of different accidents.

Foot blisters:

These are small bubble-like bumps that seem at the feet and are full of easy liquid. Some can be painless on the equal time as others are extraordinarily painful to the point of stopping you from walking or maybe make on foot difficult. They are due to friction many of the foot and socks or too much moisture from sweat or moist climate situations. Another common cause of blister formation is carrying footwear which is probably too small or tied the wrong way such that they're too tight.

The handiest way to save you blisters is to run in footwear which might be nicely ready. . A becoming walking shoe must be at least half a period large than your normal footwear considering the truth that ft swell on the equal time as you run. There ought to be room for the toe. It is also very vital to buy the right strolling socks which includes WrightSocks. These have to be manufactured from artificial cloth and not cotton as they wick away moisture from the ft consequently fending off bunching up of socks which motives blisters. The socks have to be double layered and now not have seams with a easy ground as this has a tendency to prevent blister formation due to reduced friction a few of the socks and the toes. One also can smear some petroleum jelly collectively with Vaseline on the affected regions but now not too much need for use as this may motive slipping at the identical time as going for walks.

When present method pedicure ensure the calluses are not eliminated from the toes with a razor or an emery board as they characteristic blister safety. Some runners additionally use moleskin or athletic tape over the sensitive areas which is probably more vulnerable to blister. In this case, one should make certain that the tape or moleskin is easily carried out and not the use of a wrinkles and now not too tight.

If you already have a blister or you still get a blister after strolling then it's far critical to understand how to take care of them. There are sorts of blisters; the painful type and the now not so painful type. If the blister isn't always painful it need to be left on my own for the purpose that pores and skin serves as a protective device. It ultimately bursts and drains the fluid on its personal. On the opportunity hand, if it the painful type then you can drain it themselves. This is carried out by using manner of sterilizing a needle (thru way of boiling it for 10 minutes) after which carefully piercing it. Then squeeze the liquid out and afterwards observe some antiseptic cream. Protect the region from contamination and cushion it with the aid of manner of the usage of defensive it with band-beneficial useful useful resource blister block or moleskin.

If a painful blister takes vicinity within the course of a race, one have to visit one of the clinical stations to get remedy that could help one get another time within the race with out enduring the ache.

Ankle sprains:

A sprain is an damage to a joint due to tearing of a muscle or overstretching of a ligament beyond its capability. Ankle sprains are quite not unusual even as on foot and commonly give up result from twisting or rolling of the ankle. It results in a few pain and swelling at some point of the ankle bone.

This damage is generally because of tripping or twisting which takes place at the identical time because the runner isn't always searching at or searching the road. It can display up while one steps right right right into a pothole or off a reduce and twists their ankle. It is pretty common among runners who run on tough choppy trails.

The pleasant treatment for a sprained ankle is preserving off setting any stress on it. Thus, one ought to proper now prevent strolling. An icepack allows lessen the pain similarly to carry down any swelling because of this applying some ice on the region for spherical 20 mins every five hours simply facilitates. The ankle must moreover be stored expanded and wrapped with an elastic bandage for help. Application of ice need to skip on for 2 to 3 days if the ache remains there. If the pain stops then you'll circulate lower again to a few strolling however if the swelling persists for extra than three days one need to appearance a physician to get an x-ray executed to ensure there isn't any fracturing.

Achilles tendonitis:

As the decision shows, this harm has a few element to do with the Achilles tendon. This is in which the tissues connecting the heel bone to the decrease leg muscle groups swell or end up indignant. The inform-story signs and symptoms and symptoms broaden slowly through the years and aren't without issues important. One may also experience a few pain and stiffness within the Achilles at the begin of the day which has a tendency to vanish because the day progresses or as one warms up for his or her morning run after which reappears afterwards and can also be worse than in advance than. The Achilles can also make a creaking noise whilst touched or moved.

The primary cause of this harm is too much pressure at the Achilles tendon too speedy. . The tendon becomes infected after a few tearing takes region all through diverse sports. Therefore Achilles tendonitis is because of overtraining and overexerting the frame by way of manner of the usage of taking on an excessive amount of too fast. For instance, plenty of uphill strolling can purpose this damage. Additionally, pulling down of the arch of the foot will increase hazard of developing Achilles tendonitis due to lots of stress being placed on the tendon while on foot and strolling.

The satisfactory way to save you that is avoid overstressing the Achilles tendon. Stretch in advance than walking and then hold to run at a sluggish pace and slowly boom the fee. Do no longer boom the distance you run too speedy; permit your legs to get used to a positive pace and distance earlier than moving without delay to the next diploma and do not growth extra than 10% in step with week. Do carrying occasions which incorporates toe will boom that offer a boost to the calf muscle groups and moreover upload a few unique education on the aspect of biking or swimming that allows you to supply a boost to the leg muscle companies.

The fine remedy technique is one which is composed of every rest and minimal hobby. One can deal with the harm at home and should start treatment at once after the primary ache starts offevolved. Mix rest with a few decreased interest as an excessive amount of rest can cause the joints to be stiff. Rotate the injured ankle and carry out a few calf massages and ankle stretches to make certain that there can be flexibility. If this doesn't seem to artwork then it's far vital to get professional treatment as prolonged tearing can reason tendon rupture. A health practitioner would probable advocate a quick foot insert that lifts up the heel and decreases strain on the tendon. Alternatively, a unique heel pad or cups on your taking walks footwear for cushioning the heel or a splint to be worn at night time can be used. There is also a few therapy that shall we the tendon heal and restore itself over the years.

Chapter 12: Postural Problems In The Child

Examination of a infant's spine and frightened tool can be one of the maximum important checks of their existence: the anxious device is in rate of controlling all of the abilties of our body, because it gets and sends stimuli within the shape of impulse demanding, rebalances the energy, in order that the kid can exceptional adapt to the encircling environment.

To make certain that the apprehensive device works in the correct way, it is vital that it receives correct stimulation from the receptors present for the duration of the body and, consequently, moreover inside the muscle mass that manage the posture of the neck and the backbone.

Childhood is a length of large physical hobby: jumps, competitions, falls, and injuries can cause misalignments of the spine, causing an alteration inside the functioning of the receptors and, therefore, a lower hobby of the concerned device.

In truth, if a spinal malfunction takes location, the neurons of the involved device get keep of tons much less stimulation, and the demanding device itself loses its capacity to adapt the body to environmental modifications: this will be the inspiration of a considerable weakening of the organism of the child, who ought to have an awful lot plenty less resistance to illnesses.

It may be a brilliant rule for all dad and mom to have their youngsters 's vertebral column checked as a minimum as soon as of their life, especially sooner or later of the developing years: clearly as it's far critical to observe sight, listening to and one of a kind elements on a normal foundation, a characteristic take a look at is deemed further critical of the vertebral column and of the stressful device, to repair a outstanding state of stylish health.

In truth, the pubic age, which varies from person to individual, is taken into consideration to be at immoderate hazard for the onset of vertebral deformities, every in ladies and in male subjects.

Growth and development strain the body to assume new, sometimes incorrect, positions a superb way to are looking for new balances, which, in the end, can result in incorrect attitudes of the skeleton: inside the ones times, we speak of paramorphism, indicating with this expression all that, whilst identifying an alteration of the bodily shape, it's far correctable; we talk, but, of dysmorphisms, at the equal time as skeletal adjustments have emerge as continual and can not be modified with postural re-education.

The majority of paramorphism are original in college age, frequently because of an incorrect posture took a number of the benches or to an immoderate load of backpacks and briefcases, but, if detected from the number one years of faculty, can be removed thru postural re-education; as an alternative, dysmorphisms are generated because of a lack of hobby toward paramorphism.

The most without problems verifiable paramorphism can problem the once more and the lower limbs: in flip, the former is break up into symmetrical or asymmetrical, depending on whether or not or no longer they act at the sagittal aircraft or on the frontal plane.

Among the maximum not unusual types of paramorphism we endure in thoughts:

cushty posture or asthenic dress, because of the incapacity of the body to oppose the pressure of gravity, which alters its form: the hassle suggests a head tilted in advance, a extremely good abdomen, drooping shoulders, flat ft; sooner or later, scoliotic attitudes are established; the asthenic dependancy is considered the primary purpose of the numerous paramorphism;

curved lower back and lumbar lordosis: while the dorsal physiological curve of kyphosis is more striking than everyday; there can be a bent to assess a "curved" backbone, while the attitude of curvature of the trouble recognition, inside the dorsal segment, exceeds forty °; the thoughts-set of kyphosis can be transformed, if no longer taken into consideration, into an asthenic curved lower again; collectively with the curved again, lumbar lordosis must be taken into consideration, that is fashioned as a repayment curve collectively with the remarkable belly;

scoliotic thoughts-set: in front, the vertebral column must be perfectly immediately; consequently, scoliosis is known as any deviation of the latter to the left or proper, which comes out of the vertical of the imaginary plumb line, which is going from the primary cervical vertebra to the final sacral vertebra; moreover, it become found that:

scoliosis is determined greater with out hassle within the woman intercourse than in the male, with a ratio of 3 to as a minimum one;

pleasant in the share of 25-30% it is hereditary, however, if it is gift in the same circle of relatives, it is located more often;

it may depend upon "snug" positions, which children frequently anticipate.

What makes it feasible to discover the real presence of scoliosis is the radiographic record.

However, every other technique to come across it's far to location the issue with toes collectively, in most flexion of the torso forward, with the fingers-on the feet: in case you be conscious obvious convexity at the once more (hump), we are capable of be in the presence of a scoliosis; if, rather, the rachis effects with none obvious treatment within the dorsal tract, likely, we are capable of be confronted with a easy mind-set.

The form of treatment for the scoliotic thoughts-set is associated with the severity of the alteration: as much as 30 °, it can be treated with physical workout; from 30 ° to 60 °, the use of an orthopedic help, or a corset, must be associated with bodily remedy; from 60 ° onwards, surgical treatment is usually recommended.

Diagnosis

The diagnosis is continuously medical and is finished via the statement of the affected individual or with unique instrumental exams, to recognition on the troubles and degree their quantity in every age: the observe of the affected character with a plumb line and with a postural mirror lets in to awareness on the asymmetries, deviations, and deformities; moreover, precise exams of postural reactions exist, based totally on age and maturation carried out, on the subject of the specific control structures that have interaction within the postural stability:

the sight;

the steadiness;

the automatic law of the trajectories of the actions and of the mutual articular positions of the body, thru the mechanisms of proprioception.

In the laboratory, through the digitization of information, it's far feasible to efficiently find out and degree postural troubles associated with sensible overloads on the backbone and at the limbs, within the path of sport or in uncomfortable artwork positions with:

the Posturography, to measure the imbalances within the postural system;

ground electromyography, non-invasive, for the test of electrical noise, inside the case of muscle tension;

the algometry, which specifies the amount of ache;

the inclinometer or goniometry, for the deviations of the axes of the motion;

the thermography, with which it's miles registered an boom of heat, within the case of mechanical disturbance;

ultrasound, to appearance the lesions of the entire musculoskeletal machine.

Treatment

Gymnastics and rehabilitation are the branches of rehabilitation remedy, which use motion or postures to save you and reduce the risks of mechanical alterations of the frame.

This remedy is aimed toward adults, to increase the sustainability of repetitive mechanical paintings and, therefore, to prevent or treat pain or damage to the musculoskeletal gadget; as for youngsters, as a substitute, it dreams to prevent the accumulation of microtraumas, issues or injuries, which modify the future of kids as an awful lot as deformity.

Consequently to an wrong posture, no longer best the bones, however additionally the moderate tissues assume altered states: a few muscle mass lose their tone and do now not guide the form as they must; others, on the other hand, retreat, resulting in stiff and shortened and developing sturdy tensions.

In this manner, the whole musculoskeletal device well-knownshows itself in a scenario of a strong imbalance; furthermore, it is often related to pain and beneficial headaches.

Almost commonly, postural gymnastics moreover uses respiratory gymnastics.

Who to contact

Many attempt their hand at physical bodily video games and do-it-your self sports activities, in an try and treatment the issue with out leaving home or turning to insufficient and inadequate figures, along with gyms wherein agency gymnastics takes area, jogging the risk of worsening their non-public scenario.

The maximum suitable decide to turn to is that of the posturologist: a professional within the fitness department, who has attended a path or a grasp of posturology and is, therefore, a parent that offers with diagnostics and/or postural rehabilitation, counting on the very personal specificity.

Through a particular software, the posturologist aims to re-harmonizes the musculoskeletal shape, fixing or loosening tensions and strengthening poor muscle groups, along with the abdominals.

Depending on the case, postural sports activities are used, but it moreover attracts on joint mobility, stretching, and breathing applications.

WHAT SPORT DO YOU DO FOR BACK PAIN?

What game do you do for once more pain and accurate posture?

If you have got suffered from returned ache on the identical time as soon as on your life, of direction, you may apprehend all the viable incredible treatments for this hassle, however do you furthermore can also additionally understand which sport to do for decrease once more ache?

In reality, for some time now, the first rate dependancy of the usage of game to save you and accurate any postural problems or, anyhow, to the lower back has spread.

Of direction, now not all sports sports are indicated for decrease back pain, however some are a real therapy-all and might make the difference amongst someone with the appropriate posture and one with imbalances in the spine.

Let's start from the begin.

BACK PAIN: CAUSES AND SYMPTOMS

Back pain is one of the most commonplace pain syndromes and, not quite, is one of the important motives why a medical consultation is needed.

In maximum times, it manifests itself as episodic pain of quick length, a few days or some weeks, which resolves spontaneously or with a restoration intervention of severa types.

The causes can be manifold: issues of a discopathic nature (hernias, protrusions), arthrosis, postural changes, paravertebral musculature susceptible element, muscular traumas, which consist of a stretch due to an incorrect motion or to a contracture on account of excessive stresses or incorrect postures held over the years.

In fact, we often spend hours sitting at our desks or in the car, taking positions that appear cushty to us, however which come to be risky positions for our decrease returned and which in the long run can motive imbalances, which include scoliosis, lordosis or kyphosis.

The symptom this isn't unusual to all styles of lower returned pain is a pain.

The nature of the disturbance can be successfully hooked up based totally at the right vicinity, intensity, length, and unique moments of the day in which the painful sensation occurs.

Postural treatment

Whatever the reason of back pain, the maximum indicated remedy is genuinely postural remedy.

There are numerous postural techniques and one-of-a-kind techniques utilized by professionals in the location, however all have the same goal: to rebalance the energy of the muscle businesses at the spine, freeing tensions and growing all the muscle tissues of the posterior kinetic chain, which is going from the occiput to the 'large toe.

Recommended sports activities activities and sports to avoid

To avoid once more pain, bodily interest have to be sluggish, slight, and finished correctly: due to this, it's far really helpful to be discovered at least to begin with via using an professional.

The most preferred sports sports sports activities for decrease lower again ache are:

swimming: as an interest finished in the absence of gravity, the burden of the body is decreased, and the vertebral column isn't overloaded;

on foot: it's miles a sort of interest that is beneficial for anyone and for the whole frame, but it's miles vital to take the right precautions, which consist of suitable shoes, ordinary plan, posture manage sooner or later of the journey;

pilates: facilitates each in enhancing posture and strengthening muscle tissue; Pilates is critical because of the reality the properly-being of our lower back furthermore is based upon at the muscle corporations, which need to be at the same time toned and elastic if you want to help each the steadiness and the mobility of the spine.

The sports activities to keep away from in case of lower once more pain are:

cycling, but moreover desk certain and spinning bikes;

race;

weight lifting.

These sports sports activities aren't to be condemned in an absolute way, but, putting the lumbosacral hinge and the once more in favored beneath stress, it's far higher to avoid them in order now not to strain an already inflamed place excessively.

NECK MUSCLE CONTRACTURE: SYMPTOMS, CAUSES AND REMEDIES

That of neck muscle contracture is a very disturbing and limiting circumstance in ordinary life sports activities, no matter the fact that too regularly it's far underestimated by way of individuals who be afflicted by means of it.

Neck contracture: signs and symptoms and causes

The most important symptoms of this disorder are neck ache, muscle stiffness, a experience of anxiety, heaviness, excessive problem of motion, and, in some instances, headache and dizziness.

The causes that added approximately the improvement of this hassle additionally may be severa :

overload of the neck muscle groups;

coldness;

sudden speedy and wrong movement;

incorrect postures repeated over the years;

the altered posture of the cervical tract;

discopathies (protrusions, hernias) of the cervical spine;

stress somatization, anxiety, and/or depressive states.

Neck muscle contracture treatments and remedy

It is, therefore, vital to make a differential prognosis and to select out the reason of neck pain.

Once the cause has been recognized, the maximum appropriate remedy may be directly followed, that's typically pharmacological and physiotherapeutic.

It is critical to touch a professional, which incorporates an orthopedist and/or physiatrist, who will prescribe the great and calibrated care primarily based on the specific problem and the desires of the person that suffers.

In enormous, to loosen up the muscular tissues, numerous kinds of pills are used, particularly muscle relaxants and anti-inflammatories, along the latter with instrumental healing procedures and physiotherapy manuals, in conjunction with tecar treatment, which, together with decontracting massages, are the treatments of preference, which succeed to relax and loosen up the aching muscle organizations.

The biggest and most exceptional muscle within the cervical district is in truth the trapezius muscle, which frequently goes into contracture, ensuing in the fundamental reason of neck ache.

In any case, it's miles important to take right away motion to prevent the trouble from turning into continual and growing more incapacitating secondary conditions, which, if not corrected in time and within the proper way, can emerge as everlasting, which incorporates the stiff neck, myalgia cervicalgia, postural modifications, painful shoulder, and so forth.

Chapter 13: Borne Out Of Hinduism

In the 1/3 century BC Hindu epic book of know-how, Mahabharata, monetary destroy 12, "Shanti Parva," phase on Mokshadharma, an early version of yoga named nirodhayoga modified into stated. This shape of yoga supposed, without a doubt, "yoga of cessation." This concerned an incremental withdrawal from aware concept, sensations and attention. The objective emerge as the conclusion of purusha—the higher (non secular) self. This approach involved things like vichara (which intended "diffused reflected photo") and viveka (which supposed "discrimination" or "discernment"). Some of the goals stated for yoga encompass, entering into Brahman (the super traditional precept), recognition of Brahman everywhere, setting apart actual self from the bodily realm, and masses of others. Some have said that there had been no uniform dreams for yoga due to this, but this form of claim is borne out of a lack of awareness in each of those. All of these are extremely good variations of the same cause.

Mahabharata equates yoga with Samkhya, one of the six faculties of Hindu idea—a body of expertise based on cause, precise judgment and important questioning.

The Mokshadharma section of Mahabharata includes a primitive form of meditation. With yoga, one is made able to uniting the person soul (atman) with the ideal Brahman that permeates every trouble of the universe.

The "Song of the Lord," known as the Bhagavad Gita, stays one of the more well-known factors of Mahabharata. It moreover contains a exquisite many yoga teachings. The Gita makes yoga out to be nicely matched with the ordinary sports sports of a worldly life, and not completely the province of individuals who surrender all the matters of this international.

The Gita reveals 3 key varieties of yoga:

• Jnana yoga, or the yoga of information,

• Bhakti yoga, or the yoga of devotion,

• Karma yoga, or the yoga of motion.

Made up of 18 chapters, the Gita consists of a total of 7-hundred verses (shlokas). Each financial catastrophe is marked as a separate, greater unique shape of yoga, increasing the scope of yoga's impact on our each day lives.

Throughout Hindu philosophy's maximum easy, historic sutras, yoga is cited at fantastic period. For instance, 6th to second century BC Vaisheshika sutra, of the Vaisheshika Hindu faculty, tells us that yoga is "a state in which the thoughts is dwelling high-quality in the soul and consequently no longer in the senses" (Bronkhorst).

This quotation is well matched with the cause of chickening out from all senses (pratyahara), which ends inside the cessation of all happiness (sukha) and suffering (dukkha). Beyond this, the texts communicate of similarly steps in yogic meditation that would cause the state of affairs of non secular awakening—liberation from the deterministic device of bodily truth.

In the Vedanta college of the Hindu religion, the Brahma sutras, written amongst 450 BC to AD 200, inform us that yoga is a way for reaching "subtlety of frame" and extraordinary non secular capabilities.

The Nyaya sutras (600 BC–AD hundred) speak meditation (dhyana), meditative attention (samadhi), and distinctive subjects that talk about debate, reasoning and philosophy as kinds of yoga.

Chapter 14: Beginning With Solving Your Posture

How your posture appears in recent times is not a in the destiny fault, however a surrender result of years of interest. The stress of horrible posture, over the years it can trade the anatomical tendencies of the backbone which can result in the opportunity of constricted nerves and blood vessels, further to troubles with discs, muscle organizations and joints. If you're a tall individual, perhaps you have were given humped to keep away from interest, at the same time as sitting in beauty or amongst your fellows. A brief heighted character could probable have completed a few component precisely opposite i.E. Overstretched himself to appearance taller. Both the ones situations effects in a lousy posture. Over time these terrible conduct have a protracted lasting effect upon how our posture shapes out. Our our bodies become used to the awful posture and that is why we don't even revel in any ache or pressure.

Understanding Your Posture:

The first actual step within the route of solving or improving your posture is through reading what exactly you do incorrect while repute, sitting, or taking walks. The splendid approach in the course of know-how whether your posture is correct or not is to have a observe yourself cautiously on the identical time as you stroll. Try to recognition on the frame moves from the top to toe. Also make a intellectual seen of posture and decrease back guide. A correct and fixed posture is denoted by using using cushty high-quality style of walking while an volatile posture ought to look disconnected. If you are not right at looking at the posture yourself, try asking someone else, it'll additionally assist.

Identify right posture:

What is called "suitable posture" is genuinely no longer whatever greater than keeping your frame in a immediately and aligned order. While popularity, you have got got a remarkable posture if you have a right away decrease lower back, squared shoulders, chest out, chin up and at stomach in. You have got a brilliant posture if you can draw a straight away line out of your earlobe thru your shoulder, arms, lower back, hip, knee, to the middle of your ankle.

To discover your right posture follow those few simple steps.

Mirror take a look at: Stand in the the front of mirror and align your ears, hands, shoulders, decrease returned and hips. Align your ears loosely above your shoulders and hips. These factors over again make a without delay line, however your spine itself will curves in a moderate 'S'. It appears complex but you may see that that this obtained't damage the least bit. However if if you enjoy any intense ache, then have a study your component view in a mirror to look whether or not you are forcing your again into an unnatural characteristic or no longer. If you do no longer sense any pain, it manner that your posture then need to no longer be altered, as it'd cause other problems.

Knowing the curves:

Your backbone specially has herbal curves that you need to uphold, they'll be called the 'double C' or 'S' curves, they're additionally known as lordotic and kyphotic. A lordotic curve is a curve gift in the lumbar spine, and due to the increased attitude, it is also known as lordosis of the lumbar backbone. The tremendous kyphotic curve is present in the thoracic backbone, but at the same time as this curve surpasses 50 stages it's miles known as kyphosis of the thoracic spine. Both these curves are decided from the lowest of your head for your shoulders and the curve from the pinnacle decrease again to the base of the spine. Make positive that your weight is evenly allotted, at the same time as recognition immediately for your toes. It also can experience like you are leaning in advance, or searching weird, but you aren't.

Exercises to restore your posture:

Good posture can't be done with out training your muscular tissues to do the paintings. It is giant to comply with carrying sports that red meat up the muscle mass during your higher shoulders and yet again, they help in fixing and enhancing your posture. Not continuously is growing a frame builder body a have to, building a "muscle memory" is more vital, so that you mechanically and glaringly keep or correct your posture without exhaustion. You ought to workout the agonist and antagonist muscle groups flippantly, on every occasion you workout. It technique exercising your hamstrings as plenty as your quadriceps, chest as a whole lot as your better lower decrease lower back, and so forth.

To restore your posture in widespread, strive practising theses clean physical sports at home:

Exercise One

Square your posture, have an upright head, and feature your ears aligned over your shoulders.

Palms up and along your ears enhance every hands right away out.

Bend your forearms inside the route of your shoulders, and make an effort to touch your shoulder blades collectively with your fingertips.

Do as a minimum ten repetitions with each arms, then do ten reps for every arm singularly.

Exercise Two

Follow the same alignment of ears and shoulders

Raise your palms out to facets at shoulder pinnacle, then keep for a sluggish recall of ten.

Counting to 10 as you decrease, slowly decrease fingers to the rims.

Counting to 10 as you improve hands, slowly improve arms lower lower back to shoulder height.

Do gadgets of ten, constantly checking your alignment with every rep. If twenty reps are too much for you, then try and do as many as you may. At least a moderate fatigue inside the shoulder need to be felt.

Penguin Exercise:

An exciting and clean to exercising workout is "be a penguin". Place your elbows at your facet, and speak to your shoulders together along with your each palms. Raise both elbows (rely of three) and decrease them backpedal (rely of three), at the same time as maintaining your hands to your shoulders and now have your ears aligned, do as mant reps as your body allows in the consolation vicinity. Even 30 seconds are enough for at least ten reps.

Do stretches:

If you've got got sore lower decrease lower back or neck, then this exercise can significantly help you. If your activity calls so that it will sit for long intervals, it's moreover accurate to do stretches in the course of paintings.

Stretch or tilt your head in all 4 instructions over your shoulders (left, proper, lower returned, in advance), and rub down your neck lightly. However keep away from rolling in a circle, to avoid further pressure.

Go on your knees and arms, curl your lower returned upwards, similar to a cat, and then do the alternative. Imagine approximately being capable of place a bowl within the hollow of your returned.

Repeat those few physical sports every day. Try to do them within the morning; it will assist your frame to stretch out the muscle weariness of sleep. It can also assist to elevate your electricity degree with out a heavy workout, if finished periodically in the route of the day.

Practice yoga:

Yoga is a sequence of extraordinary postures, which might be pretty good sized on your health in fashionable. Yoga allows in enhancing your balance and on foot your center muscle companies, making them stronger and assisting you to preserve a accurate body alignment. Practicing yoga might also permit you to preserve an erect posture whilst repute, sitting and strolling.

Wall take a look at:

Another commonplace way to decorate your posture is to carry out a wall test. Stand at the aspect of your head, shoulders, fingers and hips in competition to the wall and your heels about 5-6 inches ahead. Your decrease belly muscle businesses need to be drawn in and furthermore decrease the arch for your lower once more. Push yourself far from the wall and try to hold this vertical, upright alignment. It is probably your first step towards getting a exquisite posture.

Chapter 15: Daily Habits Causing Bad Posture And How To Avoid Them

Roland have grow to be a more youthful and good-looking man in his past due thirties. When he completed excessive college, he have grow to be an avid programmer due to the fact he modified into interested in pc systems. As a geek, he have turn out to be one of the brilliant programmers in his metropolis.

However, as he modified into maturing, he did refuse to workout due to the fact he felt that he become better off spending his time studying a contemporary programming language or writing a current day piece of software software. At age 35, he have end up a a success computer programmer, but he changed into a victim of lower back and neck ache. The pains have been so devastating that he often needed to take time off from work.

Sounds acquainted? I am sure anybody comprehend a person that has the identical specific complaint.

Several medical doctors accomplished numerous X-rays on Roland, however to no avail. Vinak, Roland's cousin – who is as clever and a achievement as Roland is – got down to discover the solution to his cousin's pains and to make certain that he himself, isn't vulnerable to such pain.

Vinak modified into amazed to discover that each one his cousin desires to do is to accurate a number of his postural behavior. Now Roland self warranty is renewed over again, he can now move again all over again to artwork understanding nicely that although his pains resurface over again, he is aware of what to do to them. Vinak can now take a look at the ones preventive measures to his daily physical activities just so he doesn't need to enjoy Roland's ache.

In maximum times, the idea motive of our ache lies within the each day terrible conduct which you pick out out specially in our more youthful age. It's best later that you understand the damages that those awful behavior have introduced on you; However, at that thing it might be too past due to correct them. At the time, you are trying to accurate them your frame might also moreover have grow to be too vintage to comply to new behavior.

However, there is nonetheless preference for human beings which includes you. Your conduct come to be easier to restore whilst you understand their root reason. Those conduct can without troubles be rectified in case you end up aware about them. In this financial disaster, we're going to pinpoint the proper postural conduct that purpose our pains after which what that dependancy does to our posture. So permit's start

1. Carrying a Bag On One Shoulder

When I become in excessive college, I idea that it changed into imprudent to put on baggage with each straps on. I felt that baggage that had each straps allows for a conformist, tighter posture, and constrained movement. I additionally idea that a one bag strap lets in for a swagger, much less limited and a greater comfortable motion.

But this is a bad omen.

Carrying a bag on one shoulder prevents the distribution of the burden in the frame. If you carry a heavy handbag on one shoulder, then 3 subjects are probable to take region:

Your natural gait may be thrown off.

Your muscle organizations becomes off balance.

And your muscle tissue will stiffen.

Yes, I realize that your bag is in which you maintain your basics stuffs like your cosmetics, your gym garments, your pc, your pockets, and your water bottles. However, the trouble is that the manner we have a tendency to hold our luggage round makes us slouch.

For example, If you go searching, you'll test that ladies love to carry their large luggage on one among their shoulders.

Now, I am no longer saying that sporting a bag is all that awful. I am genuinely saying that you shouldn't supply a bag on considered considered one of your shoulders mainly if you're too one-sided, or your bag affords you and not the usage of a guide.

2. Crossing legs whilst sitting

How normally have you ever ever ever crossed your legs at the place of work or at the dining table? Probably, All the time. Most people are comfortable with crossing their legs when sitting down. Those people would possibly say crossing their legs is comfortable for them.

However, I need to inform you that crossing your legs on the identical time as sitting down is a terrible pose.

It does now not simplest purpose excessive blood pressure for you, but it additionally reasons varicose veins.

The way you area your legs can distort or twist the picture human beings have approximately you.

If you aren't controlling the message in a large meeting, then it's an difficulty.

Crossing your legs for a long time frame should make your pelvis to tilt and rotate. Crossing your legs also can motive ache for your decrease again and motive misalignment of the spine, which could then purpose horrible posture

three. Cradling your cellular telephone

Many human beings don't rent headphones, due to the reality we like to cradle our telephones with our heads all the way to our shoulders. Sometimes so we get into the location in which we assist our telephones with our shoulders in desire to our palms.

Smartphone curdling is a totally excessive issue these days. Phone curdling makes our cervical backbone - this is the neck – to genuinely flex over to at least one aspect.

Since you are flexing over to at least one facet, the nerves within the bent location can turn out to be indignant. Hence, you want to save you flexing your head to at the least one side, specially in case you're maintaining it for a long time because of the reality that's going to make the nerves angry. It can also make the muscular tissues to shorten, and reason neck and shoulder ache.

4. Looking all of the way all the way down to cellphone or computer

A computer changed into designed to be cushty and available, however they're capable of motive intense pain inside the neck. Even no matter the reality that a computer is referred to as a "laptop," it isn't always designed for use on the laps. Putting a laptop to your laps exquisite forces you to slouch your head, consequently, putting large pressure on your lower back.

If you want to have a remarkable ergonomics, then constantly regulate your pc on the same time as using it. You'll be placing your neck and the extreme of your frame at danger if you're walking with a pc that is placed at the top of a table in a table or in a coffee hold.

If you go searching you in a public area, you'll see a terrific quantity of humans hunching over their smartphones. The commonplace human head weighs among 10 -12 pounds. So, consider the amount of pressure, our head puts on our neck on every occasion we slouch. We're commonly bending our necks at 60 levels on every occasion we use our phones.

5. Sitting Too Much

Today, we spend most of our lives sitting down; we sit down within the the front of our laptop table, we take a seat on the sofa while looking the extremely-contemporary episode of the NFL, We take a seat in our cars while using to artwork. Various studies has showed that we spend greater than half of of our lives sitting down.

Today, we sit for extended hours that we don't even recognise while we begin to increase terrible conduct that affect our posture.

The C-curved slouching of most workplace human beings located choppy stress on their stressful nerves and spinal discs. Because the strain compresses the inner organs, it can moreover purpose urogenital, and digestive troubles.

The pinnacle chest that results from slouching will make the diaphragm now not to absolutely descend. Slouching moreover makes the top to protrude beforehand and compress the joints some of the head and the neck which then effects in horrible recognition and tension complications.

6. Wrong Sitting

Did that your sitting function may want to make or smash your posture? Most people display off horrible horrific conduct even as sitting down. Such conduct are:

• hunching over

• leaning again

• allowing the butt to sink in

• leaning lower again

• shifting the eyeballs rather than their body

- crossing the legs

- Adjusting the seat too low

- dangling the toes

- sprawling lower back the palms on the ground

- leaning on the arms of the chair

- seating again too far inside the chair

- sitting on the desk for a long term

Now things can get lousy while you take a seat incorrectly. Since your spine is meant to aid the strain of your head closer to gravity, a few sitting positions will modify that alignment and make you slouch.

7. Driving A Car With The Other Shoulder Higher

Driving is one of the each day responsibilities, all of us do. The function of the shoulder is to offer help for the palms and save you injuries even as the usage of. Holding the steering with the right shoulder better than the opportunity shoulder can bring about horrific posture.

8. Leaning on one leg

Leaning on one leg might also seem cushty on the start, that's if you're repute for a quick time, however it can turn out to be very uncomfortable in case you intend to hold the place for a long term. Leaning on one leg forces makes you located more strain on one factor of your hip and on your decrease decrease again in place of using your middle muscle agencies and your buttocks to hold you upright.

Chapter 16: Negative Effects Of Forward Head Posture

Forward head posture can, quite, be very debilitating. It can motive persistent ache and as aforementioned, beautify into extra tough issues or conditions. If no longer fixed, the slump of the frame forward can also moreover even decrease your lung functionality as a bargain as 30%.2 Thus, it can't great purpose ache but can start to have physiological influences at the frame, disrupting normal functioning. Degenerative disc disease, osteoarthritis, herniated discs, muscle lines, headaches, thoracic outlet syndrome, sleep disruptions, and social implications are similarly troubles which could arise if postural deficits are left untreated. We explore the ones conditions and their dating to the postural imbalance called forward head posture within the sections below.

Degenerative Disc Disease

Degenerative disc disease is the damage and tear through the years of the discs placed a number of the vertebrae bones. Over 60% of the population aged 40 and over revel in a few degree of degenerative disc illness.Three The disks act as shock absorbers in the backbone, prevent painful bone-on-bone grinding and allow movement to arise in the backbone. However, as time goes on they turn out to be dehydrated and lose their cushioning capabilities. Unfortunately, not like most components of the frame, the discs are not self-repairing. They lack a right away blood deliver main to slow or no recuperation mechanisms. Symptoms of degenerative disc disease encompass, but might not be restricted to, ache inside the neck or arms, numbness or tingling inside the shoulders or fingers, loss of balance, stiffness within the neck, and in greater excessive instances, loss of bowel or bladder control because of nerve disruptions.

Forward head posture can boost up this manner. The additional weight of the top causing strain and pressure on the bones and tissues inside the neck can location pressure at the intervertebral discs, causing degeneration to stand up at a far quicker fee. Disc possibility surgical procedure does exist but is a rarity. It is a very invasive approach, and there are combined opinions on whether or now not or now not it clearly solves the problem. Many years down the line, with technological advances, this can in the end show to be a greater possible possibility. However, with the effect being moderately everlasting, posture is always substantial to save you early degeneration that would cause a domino impact of headaches and make certain accurate spinal health.

Osteoarthritis

Osteoarthritis is without delay associated with degenerative disc sickness. Similar to degenerative disc sickness, the extra weight and stress the neck endures through ahead head posture wears down the cervical backbone joints.

Osteoarthritis is a joint disease in which the cartilage in amongst joints and bones destroy down causing painful bone-on-bone touch. The cartilage on the factor joints, which can be the regions in which motion occurs within the backbone, wear down. The charge at which this takes place may be accelerated through the lack of defensive discs in many of the vertebrae. When the intervertebral discs end up degenerated, there may be a higher risk of osteoarthritis. Further, painful bone spurs, or excess boom of the bone, may also moreover increase due to the bone-on-bone grinding.

In intense instances, narrowing of the spinal wire canal can reason neurological problems affecting functioning skills. Nerves can end up compressed inflicting radiating pain and nerve signal disruptions. For example, gripping a tumbler or keeping balance have to become intricate. Other symptoms that could boom in association with osteoarthritis encompass lack of mobility inside the neck, elegant pain within the neck, neck stiffness, and sometimes, a grinding sensation at the same time as shifting the top and neck. These offer vital reasoning as to why solving in advance head posture in advance than it receives worse is crucial. Although with age and time osteoarthritis and disc degeneration can be inevitable, rushing up the machine glaringly results in useless pains and discomforts earlier on in life. Postural correction is step one in preventing early onset of osteoarthritis or exceptional spinal degeneration. Take the time to finish the right carrying activities weekly, as stated in our rehabilitation software in under. Changes won't arise right away, but over time, it's far a completely correctable situation. Through exercising, you could eliminate your neck pain and save you terrible outcomes, along side osteoarthritis, from happening.

Herniated Discs

With the lengthy-term forward positioning of the top, the vertebrae may moreover shift in advance. The mind-set at which the bones shift and the more strain created thru using the top can display and rupture intervertebral discs, maximum generally called a herniated disc.

Also known as a slipped disc, the most difficulty with this situation is that nerves in the affected vicinity can end up pinched inflicting ache, numbness, and tingling to occur. The discs placed within the cervical location are not as huge as special locations in the course of the backbone. Thus, even as a herniated disc happens, the effects and signs and symptoms may be a good buy worse. Other signs and symptoms, much like the ones of osteoarthritis and degenerative disc sicknesses, may additionally additionally encompass neck pain, ache in the shoulders and fingers, and inclined point within the neck and palms.

Conclusion

Now you've got started out your journey toward a higher, yoga lifestyles. There will although be times when you conflict, and this is in reality incredible.

Like everything else in existence – it is all about exercising. The more you exercising, the more you'll be able to think great a bit greater rationally, so you can assist diffuse a number of your stress proper now. Eventually you can get to some extent wherein you can channel any lousy energies round you into your weekly/each day yoga consultation without even pausing – but you possibly are not there yet. Keep practicing, preserve breathing, and don't overlook to center yourself.

These strategies will help you with the entirety from trekking up the stairs to calming down in advance than doing a big presentation. Remember that what you located into your frame, you may get out of it. Don't prevent moving, don't prevent pushing the limits of your body, and don't neglect that you may manipulate your happiness and usa of thoughts.